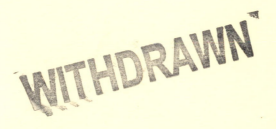

Coerced Contraception?

Hastings Center Studies in Ethics

A SERIES EDITED BY

Mark J. Hanson and Daniel Callahan

This series of books, published by The Hastings Center and Georgetown University Press, examines ethical issues in medicine and the life sciences. Established in 1969, The Hastings Center, located in Briarcliff Manor, New York, is an independent, nonprofit, and nonpartisan research organization. The work of the Center is mainly carried out through research projects, the publication of the *Hastings Center Report* and *IRB: A Review of Human Subjects Research*, and numerous workshops, conferences, lectures, and consultations. **The Hastings Center Studies in Ethics** series brings the ongoing research of The Hastings Center to a wider audience.

Coerced Contraception?

Moral and Policy Challenges of Long-Acting Birth Control

EDITED BY
Ellen H. Moskowitz
Bruce Jennings

GEORGETOWN UNIVERSITY PRESS / WASHINGTON, D.C.

Georgetown University Press, Washington, D.C. 20007
© 1996 by Georgetown University Press. All rights reserved.
10 9 8 7 6 5 4 3 2 1   1996
THIS VOLUME IS PRINTED ON ACID-FREE ∞ OFFSET BOOK PAPER

Library of Congress Cataloging-in-Publication Data

Coerced contraception? : the moral and policy challenges of long-
   acting birth control / edited by Ellen H. Moskowitz, Bruce
   Jennings.
          p.   cm.—(Hastings Center studies in ethics)
      1. Birth control—Moral and ethical aspects. 2. Birth control—
   Moral and ethical aspects—United States. 3. Contraceptives—Moral
   and ethical aspects. 4. Social policy—Moral and ethical aspects.
   5. United States—Social policy—Moral and ethical aspects.
   I. Moskowitz, Ellen H.   II. Jennings, Bruce, 1949– .   III. Series.
   HQ766.15.C64   1997
   363.9′6—dc20
   ISBN 0-87840-624-7 (cloth)   96-11859

Contents

Introduction

In December 1990 the United States Food and Drug Administration approved the contraceptive Norplant. It is a highly effective birth control method, consisting of six small hormone-releasing rods that are inserted in a woman's upper arm and last up to five years. Norplant was the first wholly new contraceptive option to become available in the United States since the pill's introduction in 1960. After nearly twenty-five years of research, including clinical trials involving 55,000 women in forty-four countries, and after some 500,000 had already used the method worldwide, American women had a new and different birth control alternative.

To many, Norplant seemed like a welcome addition to women's contraceptive options and choices, and it quickly caught on in the United States. Nationwide, Norplant was soon eligible for state Medicaid coverage. Private sales exceeded projections during the first year despite its relatively high initial cost, which was in the $500 to $1000 range.

However, the honeymoon with Norplant was short-lived. It was soon embroiled in a thicket of controversy. A few months after the FDA approval, a California judge presiding over a case of a woman convicted of criminal child abuse had imposed implantation with Norplant in lieu of a lengthy prison sentence. That ruling attracted national media attention. Shortly thereafter, a bill was introduced in the Kansas legislature that offered women on welfare a cash bonus if they agreed to use the contraceptive. Other states began to look at similar measures as well as laws to require Norplant use for women convicted of drug charges.

Outside of the criminal justice and social welfare context, the issue of teens using Norplant also caught the public eye. Public health officials in Baltimore made that city the focus of controversy when they announced plans to add Norplant to existing school-based reproductive health services and proposed to pilot test the program in one predominantly African-American high school. Even before the program could be implemented, it came under attack. Although many parents and students at the school favored the plan, some local clergy and community leaders mounted a protest campaign against it, expressing concerns about the health effects of Norplant, the morality of teen contraception, and the motives of city officials. While some saw in Norplant an important benefit to women, others saw it as a corrupting influence and a tool of manipulation and oppression.

Norplant is just one in a series of drugs and modalities of delivery that are revolutionizing long-term contraception. In 1992, the FDA approved Depo-Provera, a three-month hormonal method that is administered by injection. In the late 1980s the intrauterine device Copper-T 380A became available in the United States, and it was recently determined to remain effective for up to ten years. A new generation of hormone-releasing IUDs will soon be available. Other technologies, such as contraceptive vaccines, long-acting hormone-releasing vaginal rings, and new forms of implant systems and injectables may reach U.S. markets within the next ten years.

How will our society cope with reversible, long-term birth control? There are no easy answers. These contraceptives have a socially and ethically double-edged quality. They present a method of administration that is relatively noninvasive, at least as compared with surgical sterilization, currently the most widely used form of birth control among men and women in the United States. They carry low levels of medical risk, require minimal medical supervision, and do not require a direct decision or action by either partner each day or during each act of intercourse.

In one sense, all these features make a long-acting contraception a boon, particularly to women, that greatly enhances reproductive freedom by removing most of the practical obstacles that have hindered many women from using contraceptive methods effectively in the past. Neither foresight nor a daily dosage regime—nor indeed any special attention or self-consciousness about contraception at all—is required. And unlike condoms, women need not obtain the cooperation or assent of their male partners. Long-acting methods can remove the burden—and the responsibility—of continuous choice.

Ironically, it is precisely this safety, reversibility, and convenience that create the possibility that long-acting contraception could significantly restrict the reproductive freedom of some women. These features also make it attractive to some as a tool of social policy—that is, as a means to address complex, severe, and seemingly intractable problems such as child abuse and intergenerational poverty.

Will these technologies enhance freedom of reproductive choice or become potent new instruments of coercive social control? In what way do questions of race, class, gender, and power intertwine when long-acting contraceptives are seen as the behavioral tools of social welfare, public health, and child protection policies? Should the use of contraception ever be mandatory, and how would such a requirement be enforced? Should contraception always be a woman's or a couple's free choice, and if so, what does that mean in practice? As policies are developed to encourage the use of these methods, how does one analyze the line separating ethically illicit coercion from pressures, inducements, incentives, and persuasion designed to obtain a woman's voluntary consent?

The purpose of this volume is to identify and assess the moral and policy challenges posed by long-acting contraception. Prompted by the extent to which long-term methods, particularly Norplant, have aroused controversy and suspicion, these essays aim to provide carefully reasoned and multidisciplinary perspectives on the ethical and social dilemmas these technologies raise.

The papers collected here grew out of a two-year Hastings Center project, "The Ethics of Long-Term Contraception: Ethical Guidelines for Public Policy," supported by the Ford Foundation and the Rockefeller Foundation. Between 1992 and 1994, health care professionals, ethicists, reproductive rights activists, lawyers, and social scientists joined with Hastings Center staff to consider moral and policy challenges raised by long-acting contraceptives. Over the course of four extended conferences, as well as during many informal meetings and conversations, our diverse research group identified points of difference as well as agreement. Although the work focused primarily on the United States, we also included an important international component centered on developing countries. This prolonged period of study, punctuated by lively, sometimes heated exchanges, gave thorough hearing to a broad range of pressing and complex ethical, social, and legal issues surrounding long-acting contraception and public policy.

The papers in this volume have been grouped into four sections, which reflect the scope of our deliberations. Part I contains the report and recommendations from the project. This paper provides an overview of the ethical issues in several different clinical and policymaking settings. It offers our own framework for analyzing these issues and proposes specific guidelines for clinical counseling practice and public policy.

Part II provides a historical and scientific background with which one can better comprehend the current controversies surrounding long-term contraceptives. Kathleen Powderly begins by highlighting important developments in the history of the American birth control movement, starting with the late nineteenth century. She suggests that contemporary conflicts surrounding long-term contraception are but one example of an enduring tension between salutary efforts to empower women to control their fertility and eugenic practices to limit the fertility of poor women and women of color. George Brown focuses on the history of the long-term methods themselves, characterizing their development as linked to the demographic perspective that has motivated many programs in international family planning. He explores the effects of the lengthy, complex, often uncertain processes by which new contraceptives are developed and introduced and outlines several long-acting methods which are likely to become available in the next ten years.

A number of alternative conceptual and theoretical frameworks are explored in part III. Several of these discussions center on how best to understand autonomy and coercion in reproductive decisions and how to understand the ethical responsibilities that contraceptive and reproductive choices entail. Bonnie Steinbock examines long-term contraceptives from the perspective of coercion, arguing that it is often far from clear whether a given policy or program is coercive because the concept is complex and often difficult to apply. She finds that while analysis from the perspective of coercion can provide important insight, it must be used with care lest overuse blind critics to other grounds of moral analysis. John Robertson develops the theme of reproductive responsibility and focuses on the ethical limits government bodies face in crafting policies that limit reproduction based on this rationale. Rooting his analysis in the moral and constitutional right of procreation as well as the distinctive features of Norplant, he urges government bodies to eschew such policies unless they incorporate voluntary choice.

John Arras and Jeffrey Blustein also scrutinize long-term contraception through the lens of reproductive responsibility, providing an account of the nature and grounds of the concept. They conclude that reproductive responsibility is a useful device for moral assessment and defensible against those who would argue for a notion of unfettered reproductive choice. However, they also outline its limits, particularly when the concept is looked to as a sufficient justification for a variety of troubling social policies.

Rebecca Dresser zeroes in on the problem of long-term contraception in the criminal justice system. Highlighting the ethical and policy dimensions raised by employing these contraceptives as punishment, she concludes that in some cases they can comprise a morally legitimate component of a criminal sentence and proposes a method by which they might be offered. Finally, Hilde Lindemann Nelson and James Lindemann Nelson detail how feminist theory provides special resources for exploring the ethics of using long-acting contraceptives to shape social policy. In so doing they address the fact of many strains of feminist theory and describe a distinctive theoretical impulse that they believe characterizes the varying approaches.

Part IV turns to some of the particular concerns raised by long-acting contraceptives in developing countries. This section begins with an essay by Ruth Macklin. Drawing upon insights gained while at work on reproductive ethics and health in China, Mexico, and the Philippines, she argues that cultural values play a more limited role in influencing a woman's decision whether to use a long-term contraceptive than is ordinarily thought to be the case. Macklin proposes that a woman's social and economic class, her nation's specific government policies, the practices of her health care providers, and the degree of freedom from control she has from her sexual partner are key determinants for behavior. Tola Olu Pearce then explores ethical problems raised by the importation of long-acting contraceptives into Nigeria. Her examination distinguishes factors arising at the global, national, and household levels. The challenges posed by long-term contraceptives in Brazil and the Dominican Republic are analyzed by Ellen Hardy. She suggests that the unique advantages of these methods have also been the source of ethical problems—problems rooted in inadequate political and financial support by government agencies, inadequate access to health information and care, and tensions between the desire to offer these methods and the potential for abuse.

The editors are indebted to the project's co-director, Daniel Callahan, and to our core research group, who gave generously of their time and were instrumental in making this project so productive: John D. Arras, Karen J. Beattie, George F. Brown, Irene W. Crowe, Rebecca Dresser, Jacqueline Darroch Forrest, Willard Gaylin, Lila G. Gracey, Jane M. Johnson, Patricia A. King, Luella Klein, Ruth Macklin, Luz Alvarez Martinez, Hilde Lindemann Nelson, James Lindemann Nelson, Rosalind Petchesky, Cheri Pies, Kathleen E. Powderly, John A. Robertson, Allan Rosenfield, Julia R. Scott, and Bonnie Steinbock.

We also thank the following individuals who aided our effort by participating in project meetings or otherwise rendering much valued assistance: Charon Asetoyer, Alberta Arthurs, Peter Beilenson, Jerry Bennett, David G. Blankenhorn, Jeffrey Blustein, Martha Brady, Lybia Burgos, Davy Chikamata, Cynthia B. Cohen, Juan Diaz, Jennifer Frost, John Gill, Sarah Gill, Ellen Hardy, Margaret L. Hempel, Jane Hughes, Joanne Hustead, Lisa Kaeser, Cynthia Klaisle, Marion T. Leyds, Elizabeth Miola, Penda N'Diaye, Tola Olu Pearce, Michael Policar, Margaret Polaneczky, Philip R. Reilly, Steven W. Sinding, Melody Smith, Joanne Spicehandler, Lynn Szwaja, and Alan Wolfe.

This project was made possible by grants from the Ford Foundation and the Rockefeller Foundation, and we are grateful for their support. Another outcome of the project, *Long-Acting Contraception: Moral Choices, Policy Dilemmas*, was published as a special supplement to the *Hastings Center Report* 25, no. 1 (1995): S1-S32, and has been widely disseminated to government officials and health care providers. The supplement contains the full text of part I, chapter 1 and short versions of each chapter of part II and part III of this book. Part I, chapter 2, by John A. Robertson, is a modified version of chapter 4 of John A. Robertson's *Children of Choice: Freedom and the New Reproductive Technologies* (Princeton: Princeton University Press, 1994, copyright© 1994 by Princeton University Press), reprinted here with the permission of the author and Princeton University Press.

ELLEN H. MOSKOWITZ
BRUCE JENNINGS

PART I: Overview and Guidelines

ELLEN H. MOSKOWITZ, BRUCE JENNINGS, AND
DANIEL CALLAHAN

Long-Acting Contraceptives: Ethical Guidance for Policymakers and Health Care Providers

Ellen H. Moskowitz, Bruce Jennings, and
Daniel Callahan

Long-Acting Contraceptives: Ethical Guidance for Policymakers and Health Care Providers

In recent years, medicine has offered American women a new generation of safe, reversible, and highly effective long-acting contraceptives. Since 1988 two new types of intrauterine devices (IUDs) have become available—the Copper-T 380A, known by its trade name, Paragard, which provides up to eight years of contraceptive effect, and a one-year IUD, sold under the name Progestasert, which works by releasing the hormone progesterone. In 1990 the federal Food and Drug Administration (FDA) approved Norplant, a six-rod subcutaneous implant that releases the synthetic hormone progestin and lasts up to five years. Two years later the FDA approved depot medroxyprogesterone, known by its trade name, Depo-Provera, a three-month progestational method administered by intramuscular injection.

The advent of effective, long-acting contraception should be welcome. Individual birth control preferences vary from person to person and in the same person over time. Increased birth control options improve the likelihood of user satisfaction and effective contraceptive use. However, the social reception of these new methods, particularly the widely publicized Norplant, has been mired in controversy, suspicion, and even ethnic conflict. Instead of being seen as one means for enhancing reproductive choice, long-term methods have been viewed as instruments of gender or racial discrimination and tools for limiting personal control. Instead of being regarded as a needed corrective to our nation's unsatisfactory—even substandard—current approach to the serious problem of unintended pregnancy among women of all ages and backgrounds—and one particularly well-suited to individuals who have difficulty with the active, daily regimens of oral contraceptives and barrier methods, long-term contraceptives have been dismissed by some as instruments of class prejudice and eugenic social coercion.

An understanding of this discord rests on certain facts and ethical principles. Among the central factual concerns are the intrinsic properties of available long-term methods which lend themselves to surveillance and monitoring by second parties. It is also important to regard the seemingly intractable, wrenching societal problems of criminal child abuse and multigenerational poverty as well as the fact that this country has endured and continues to struggle with discrimination on the basis of class, race, and gender. The key normative concepts are freedom and coercion.

We go on to propose that unnecessary conflict and confusion result from judging policies about long-acting contraceptives strictly in terms of an absolute contrast between liberty or coercion. Our essential complaint is that the approach vastly oversimplifies the complexity of contraceptive decision making in the real lives of women and men and the difficult choices often posed in a clinical setting. As a conceptual framework for debate at the public policy level, this approach feeds our divisions and undermines our connections.

Rather than base ethical analysis on this divide, we propose facing more squarely the fact that contraceptive decisions necessarily occur in the context of relationships, not in a vacuum. The lens of freedom and coercion is unhelpful as well as divisive, blinding us to important relational realities. It is also morally unattractive. We outline an alternative perspective for grappling with ethical issues raised by long-acting contraceptives that takes fuller account of the social dimension of reproduction and contraceptive decision making.

Finally, we conclude by setting forth selected guidelines for policymakers and health care providers that express this alternative perspective. The guidelines address some of the more vexing ethical issues that these methods have presented. While our alternative method has often led us to make recommendations similar to those that might result from a freedom vs. coercion inquiry, in select instances—most notably involving directive counseling to use long-term methods—our conclusions do differ.

From Potential Promise to Perceived Threat

The long-term contraceptives developed thus far do not permit women to immediately initiate and discontinue use by their own actions: all rely on health care providers for initiation, and users cannot discontinue their contraceptive effect without substantial delay or professional assistance. Norplant and IUDs require a visit to a health care provider for insertion and removal. Depo-Provera is initiated by health provider injection, and while discontinuing it requires no second-party intervention, women must wait months for the last injection to dissipate. These contraceptives offer good opportunities for second parties to monitor a woman's period of infertility and to be confident that she is indeed infertile. While permanent sterilization offers the same opportunities, other reversible contraceptives—for example, condoms, diaphragms, or oral contraceptives—do not.

The fact that long-acting contraceptives are supervised by a second party has led some to view the methods as means of addressing some complex and severe problems—problems involving palpable human tragedy that seem unresolvable by traditional approaches such as prison terms, psychological counseling, unconditioned public assistance, and remedial education. For example, in the hope of addressing child abuse, some judges have devised probation arrangements that require the use of Norplant.[1] Seeking to decrease reliance on welfare, a number of state legislators have introduced, but not yet passed, bills requiring women who receive public assistance to accept Norplant implants.[2] To address teenage pregnancy, some have supported making Norplant an attractive contraceptive option for poor adolescents by providing it at little or no cost in school-based clinics.[3]

Similar issues are arising at the clinical level. For example, providers sometimes serve clients who are unable to successfully use oral contraceptives or barrier methods yet appear currently unready to take on the responsibilities of parenthood. Rather than simply prescribing another cycle of pills and awaiting the next abortion or child welfare crisis, some providers may instead try to encourage the use of Norplant, Depo-Provera, or an IUD. If the client wants to discontinue Norplant or an IUD, the providers may resist those requests or attempt to change the client's mind.

These kinds of policies and clinical practices have led to charges of coercion and the violation of individual reproductive freedom. The argument runs as follows: individuals have a fundamental right to control whether they will have children, and neither the government nor any individual is entitled to shape or influence a woman's contraceptive choices. This view rests on values of personal autonomy, bodily integrity, competency, and privacy. Because decisions to use long-acting contraceptives involve and may affect these values and interests, individual women have the right to make these decisions free from undue influence by others. Attempts to affect contraceptive behavior should not extend beyond neutral, nondirective education about the technological nature and physiological consequences of different contraceptive options. Also, the private, intimate nature of sexuality and reproduction renders all outside influence suspect.

This critical, suspicious response to Norplant and other long-acting methods also reflects deep worries about discrimination in the United States on the basis of class, race, and gender. These worries are not unreasonable. To a significant degree we are a country divided as well as enriched by our differences. We remain afflicted by persistent discrimination against the poor, persons who are members of racial and ethnic minorities, and women. Also, the United States has a sorry history of imposing permanent contraception, in the form of sterilization, on socially marginal, stigmatized, or disabled persons. From the 1920s to the 1950s, eugenic sterilizations were increasingly common, supported by the laws of most states, federal constitutional law, private eugenics groups, and some individual medical practitioners. The goal was purportedly to improve national life by preventing certain classes of people, often women who were poor and of non-European descent, from having children.[4]

An Alternative View

We find these concerns valid and understandable. But we do not believe that they provide a sufficient basis for ruling out any and all goals other than individual reproductive freedom in the area of contraceptive access and education. In fact, seeing these facts through the lens of freedom and coercion has unnecessarily amplified the strife surrounding the long-acting methods— so much so that the contraceptives' potential for good has been undermined. We offer a different method for thinking about the long-term methods— namely, that all influences to use long-acting contraceptives are not necessarily unethical and coercive. Such influences are ubiquitous and inevitable. They should not be dismissed or mindlessly attacked, but examined carefully on a case-by-case basis. Some will be justifiable. The guiding idea that is most helpful is not an absolutist conception of individual reproductive rights but a conception of responsible decision making in the context of relationships. True reproductive freedom is best understood not as an unequivocal right of noninterference, but rather as set within relationships of involvement and influence—concern and respect—with others.

There is a strong social as well as individual dimension of reproduction and thus of contraceptive decision making. Sexuality and reproduction are never solely self-regarding and merely private. They always have both social consequences and social dimensions. Some of these involve close relationships with others such as sexual partners, family, and close friends. Other relationships are actually quite distant—for example, those involving health care providers, religious leaders, and community leaders. An individual may be directly affected by strong cultural and religious norms that affect intimate details of behavior about sexuality and procreation.

The web of relationships that comprise reproduction and contraceptive decision making—particularly those relationships with sexual partners and children—creates responsibilities. Contraceptive choices should be guided by these responsibilities as well as by individual rights and interests. Furthermore, it is possible to consider both individual interests and the interests of others: the two are not necessarily opposed.

It is also important not to lose sight of the fact that unwanted, mistimed pregnancies can directly and foreseeably harm the pregnant woman as well as others to whom the woman has responsibilities. Women continue to be most responsible for the considerable and demanding daily activities of child rearing; consequently, unwanted and mistimed pregnancies can substantially limit a woman's opportunities to shape her life in accord with her own needs and goals, including opportunities for education, income, and satisfying marriage and parenthood. It can also upset existing relationships and harm other persons, particularly vulnerable, dependent children. Refraining from procreation in order to prevent initial or additional childbearing, or to space births, can substantially contribute to a better quality of life for an individual woman and for others close to her.

Two important conclusions follow and should guide both public policies and clinical practices concerning long-acting contraceptives. First, access to a range of effective contraceptives, including the new long-acting methods, is critically important: reproductive freedom and responsibility depend on effective choices. Second, in some cases it can be reasonably foreseen that unwanted, mistimed pregnancy will cause substantial harm. In a subset of these cases, it will be reasonable to judge that if a woman is not provided with access to a long-term method, and if she does not give serious thought to using this particular type of contraceptive, her own interests will be compromised, and so will the interests of others to whom she owes responsibilities, particularly her dependent children.

In other words, there are two equally significant ethical risks associated with long-acting contraceptives, not just one. One risk, which has received most public attention, is that women will be improperly or unjustly influenced to use the methods. The second is the risk of *mistaken or improperly influenced nonuse*. In these instances it can be appropriate and responsible to use different techniques to influence a woman to consider long-term contraceptive use, even if she is not immediately inclined to do so. Under the proper circumstances, this influence can demonstrate the best kind of care, commitment, and respect. Furthermore, abdicating this involvement in the name of individual reproductive freedom can amount to a wrongful disregard of the interests and well-being of others.

Accepting this possibility of justifiable influence requires appreciating the limits of any single individual's knowledge, perspective, and life circumstances. Effective autonomy is partly a function of age and experience. Possessing greater maturity than adolescents, adults can be prudent and ethically appropriate sources of guidance. The prudent exercise of reproductive freedom does not take place in a social vacuum, and coercive background circumstances are just as morally troubling as are coercive interpersonal pressures.

For example, adult counseling and influence are not the only forces impinging on a teen's decision to become sexually active. A surrounding environment of peer pressure, erotic symbolism, and the psychological need for acceptance, love, and self-esteem can put individual teens at tremendous risk of an unwanted or ill-timed pregnancy. It is shortsighted to focus on counseling regarding contraception as the single—or even the most powerful—coercive influence in an adolescent woman's life.

Counselors clearly should give accurate, complete information about contraception. But they need not always adopt the stance of so-called nondirective counseling. Value-neutrality is more illusory than real or respectful here: serious discussions of long-term contraceptive choices sometimes must be value-laden, covering the teen's own current and future interests as well as the interests of others to whom they now owe, and will in the future owe, responsibilities.

The possibility of justifiable influence is not limited to adolescents. Occasionally, an adult will also be unprepared to make a contraceptive choice that furthers her interests and satisfies her responsibilities based solely on a nondirective, seemingly value-neutral listing of available contraceptive options. In some cases she too will benefit from the more involved aid and guidance of others.

At bottom, the question is not whether a woman's judgment and decisions about long-acting contraceptives are influenced by others, but whether they are influenced in a fair, sound, and justifiable way. We have suggested that this requires a close, particularized, case-by-case analysis that has a richer focus than is possible within the exclusive framework of freedom and coercion. More telling and helpful is to consider a broader range of factors such as (1) the individual and relational interests at stake; (2) the need for access; (3) the possibility of mistaken nonuse as well as mistaken use; and (4) the biases and power imbalances that characterize our past history and current circumstances, particularly as expressed in reproductive matters.

Guidelines for Policymakers and Health Care Providers

Selected guidelines that express this orientation follow. The guidelines focus on what we believe to be particularly vexing ethical issues that these methods present to both policymakers and health care providers. The first part addresses policymakers, including legislators, judges, and administrators in government and nongovernment agencies involved in reproductive health. The second part concerns health care providers.

Policymakers

1. Access. *Long-acting contraceptives should be available at a fair price for informed, voluntary use by women in the United States, regardless of income or age. This requires health insurance and service delivery systems that make these methods available along with the entire range of safe and effective contraceptives and that also address the methods' special characteristics, particularly the need for removal by health care providers. Policymakers ought to develop service delivery plans, written protocols, and oversight practices that ensure appropriate access. This may include efforts to direct additional resources to reach women in special circumstances, such as adolescent mothers, where evidence strongly demonstrates that encouraging use of a long-acting method will be beneficial.*

Fair Pricing.   Access depends on fair pricing. In the United States, Norplant kits, including the implants and insertion materials, have been sold by the pharmaceutical company Wyeth-Ayerst Laboratories for approximately $365, a high initial lump-sum cost as compared with other contraceptives. Moreover, the company has failed to follow the common practice of offering the contraceptive at a lower cost to public sector providers. Because of the need to have a small stockpile of devices on hand and because Medicaid reimbursement is so low, many clinics serving low-income populations find it very difficult to offer this new contraceptive to the women who request it. Also, for low-income women not eligible for Medicaid, these costs present a substantial barrier to use. The development of Norplant did not represent an enormous initial investment in research and development for Wyeth-Ayerst. Its development and testing were supported by the federal government and private foundations, including a nonprofit organization, the Population Council.[5] The current pricing structure of Wyeth-Ayerst is questionable and should be changed to facilitate access.

Insurance Coverage.   Because of the relatively high price of long-acting contraceptives, appropriate access to the methods will often depend on insurance coverage. Current health insurance for contraception fails to accomplish this goal satisfactorily. First, too many women lack any health insurance, whether private or public.[6] Second, even if women have private-sector insurance, it is more likely than not that their policy provides no routine coverage for any reversible contraceptive, including long-acting methods. This should be changed. These methods have a legitimate place in a comprehensive approach to reproductive health services and should be included in insurance coverage for these services. It is worth noting that in cases where women have public or private insurance coverage for Norplant or IUDs at the time of insertion, they risk being uninsured when they wish removal.[7] Financial guarantees of removal should be extended at the time of insertion for any long-acting method requiring provider removal. Finally, in cases where removals are ostensibly covered by insurance, reimbursement is sometimes subject to insurers' restrictions, such as the existence of a "medical reason" for discontinuation. Insurance coverage of removals should be unconditional.[8]

Service Delivery Systems.   Taken by itself, access to long-acting methods is an incomplete ethical objective; the services to which access is secured must themselves be of high quality. The safe and respectful use of Norplant, in particular, places substantial demands on the infrastructure of health services in a woman's community for appropriate counseling, skillful insertion and removal, and appropriate follow-up care. Regions lacking a suitable service delivery system are not competent to offer these methods and should not do so. For example, in light of the continuing effect of long-term methods, a suitable service delivery system must provide continuing access to care and supervision, not simply access to insertion and removal. Women must be able to consult health care providers about their medical questions or complaints they believe are linked to the action of the contraceptives. Other necessary elements include the availability of a variety of contraceptives, not just long-term methods, and sufficient numbers of health care personnel trained and competent in counseling about the new methods in ways that demonstrate respect, care, and support for each client. Sufficient numbers of providers must also be proficient in the initiation, follow-up, and discontinuation of the methods.

Adolescents.   It is particularly important that sexually active teenagers not be denied appropriate access to long-acting contraceptives. Compared with other developed countries, United States adolescents have similar levels of sexual activity, lower levels of sex education and contraceptive use, and higher levels of unintended pregnancy.[9] One important public health response is to improve adolescents' education about and access to long-acting methods. For example, research shows that the selection of Norplant by adolescent mothers as a method of contraception is associated with higher rates of continued use and lower rates of new pregnancy than the selection of oral contraceptives.[10] In contrast, another recent study examined whether providing adolescent mothers with enhanced family planning services would delay future childbearing. The teenage mothers were not offered long-acting contraceptives, but they received wide-ranging services, including case managers trained to work with teenage parents and workshops on parenting skills, contraceptive methods, and sexually transmitted diseases. The girls were counselled about employment and education possibilities and were offered on-site Graduate Educational Development (GED) courses. They also attended classes on how to delay repeat pregnancies, plan future childbearing, and develop general life and family management skills. They were offered child care and transportation to classes, and those who failed to attend a substantial number of educational and counselling activities lost a portion of their monthly welfare grant. Despite these efforts, the researchers concluded the enhanced services did little or nothing to delay subsequent pregnancies.[11]

As with adults, appropriate access requires adherence to principles of informed consent and confidentiality. Policies should not condition an adolescent's use of a long-term method on parental consent or notification if the adolescent is capable of providing informed consent to the contraceptive.[12]

Baltimore is experimenting with school-based clinics that offer contraceptives or referrals for contraceptives as a part of primary health care, including long-term methods, and other communities may follow suit. Such experiments are reasonable and appropriate, but require sensitive planning and implementation in light of the mandatory nature of school attendance and the differing attitudes in the community about teenage sexuality. One important element is the participation of adolescents, their parents, and other interested persons in system design, monitoring, and redesign.

2. Public Assistance. *Public assistance payments for persons of low income should not be conditioned or affected by the use of long-acting contraceptives. This wrongly influences use.*

Driven by poor economies and the need to cut back state government budgets, selected officials and their constituents have increasingly come to demand a clear connection between public expenditures and outcome. One government program attracting particular scrutiny is public assistance for the poor. Increasingly, state legislatures have proposed using public assistance payments as levers to exact a certain accountability from recipients. For example, in Ohio and Wisconsin persons dependent on welfare now risk losing state subsidies if they fail to prevent their children's truancy from school. Colorado and Maryland reduce payments to parents who neglect to have their children immunized. In Arkansas, Georgia, and New Jersey, public welfare monies are not increased to cover the added expenses incurred by families who have additional children while receiving public assistance.[13]

As part of this trend, a number of state legislatures are considering using public assistance payments as levers to encourage women welfare recipients to avoid childbearing by using long-acting contraception.[14] This is inappropriate for a number of reasons. Mandating the use of long-acting contraceptives is an invasive act that violates the integrity of the physician-patient relationship. A woman's health may make it physically dangerous for her to use a hormonal method, or she may be unable to tolerate the side effects for a variety of personal, social, or cultural reasons. Her local health care system may lack personnel with adequate training and expertise in the long-acting methods. She may be celibate or perfectly happy with her current method and competent in its use. Furthermore, although she receives public assistance, she may wish to have a child and be quite capable of providing the child with good care. Yet these public assistance proposals would have this woman adopt a method that offers no benefit to her (except cash), but poses burdens involved in its use. Included in these burdens is the demeaning result of effectively paying a woman to take a particular course of action about her fertility, contraceptive use, and childbearing. The approach offends strong, widely held norms on the noncommercial nature of sexuality and reproduction.

3. Child Abuse. *Avoiding incarceration for child abuse should not be conditioned on the use of long-acting contraceptives. This wrongly influences use.*

As the criminal justice system struggles with insufficient resources, policy-makers are focusing increased attention on alternatives to incarceration such as electronic monitoring in the home and supervised community service.[15] Another approach under consideration is to condition probation for women convicted of child abuse on the use of long-acting contraceptives, especially Norplant. Although no state legislature has yet codified this scheme, growing numbers of judges have tried it.[16]

While family planning counseling, including discussions about long-acting contraceptives, may be appropriate for these women, they should not be forced to face the alternative of long-term contraception or prison. Even apart from serious questions of constitutionality, this policy direction unwisely involves the state in relying on a heavy-handed influence (the threat of incarceration) to bring about two sensitive consequences: a bodily invasion and a particular action with respect to fertility.[17] The criminal justice system should not bluntly drive a class of women to use a specific medical technology that enters the body and is accompanied by certain physiological risks, some more serious in certain women. Neither should the criminal justice system pointedly influence substantial numbers of diverse women to choose a single course of action about private matters of fertility, contraceptive use, and childbearing. This transgresses sound limitations on state intrusions in reproductive matters.[18]

In light of these problems, it is important to refrain from undertaking this new policy until and unless there is solid evidence demonstrating the policy's advantages over current or alternate approaches not subject to these faults. Simply because a woman may be guilty of child abuse, it does not follow that either the protection of others in her care or her own rehabilitation will be served by this contraceptive technology. No persuasive evidence suggests that use of a long-acting contraceptive will rehabilitate criminal offenders, deter their future criminal acts, or deter the criminal acts of others.

4. Research Directions. *Government and nongovernment agencies that finance contraceptive research should use their grant-making powers to improve access to a broader range of contraceptives.*

Male Contraceptives.   There is a pressing need for a range of male contraceptives, including long-acting, reversible methods. Owing perhaps in some measure to gender bias as well as to technical biological difficulties posed by the male reproductive system, the development of male contraceptive methods has lagged behind female methods. Although the male reproductive biology is more difficult to interrupt, part of the lack of past research can be attributed to a fear of affecting the male libido—a fear unmatched by a similar concern with the female libido.

Protection Against Sexually Transmitted Diseases.   The rising incidence of sexually transmitted diseases, particularly the deadly virus that causes AIDS, calls for the development of contraceptives that protect against these diseases, as well as interventions that provide safeguards against disease without contraceptive effect.

User Control. The existing long-acting methods do not permit women to immediately initiate or discontinue the methods by their own actions. Research is needed to develop a range of long-acting methods that enhance user control. This will depend on careful attention to the diversity of potential users' preferences and circumstances. For example, sometimes user control is best met by a long-acting method that depends on regular provider involvement: given a woman whose sexual partner or family strongly objects to her use of contraceptives, an injection of Depo-Provera may further her interest in individual control to a greater degree than a barrier method.

Health Care Providers

5. Provider-Dependent Discontinuation. *Patients who use long-acting contraceptives dependent on provider intervention for discontinuation must have ready access to removal. In the process of obtaining informed consent for removal, providers should discuss the pros and cons of that decision with care and respect. Providers should accede to the patient's settled resolve to remove or discontinue use of a long-acting contraceptive.*

Ready Access to Removal.   Appropriate use of Norplant and IUDs depends on ready access to provider removal. This means that initial counselling about these methods must cover how patients will obtain financial and clinical access to removals. It also means that health care providers who initiate these devices are under a continuing obligation to their patients to remove the devices.

Informed Consent to Removal.   Ready access to removal does not prevent health care providers from probing or questioning a removal request for the purpose of satisfying requirements of informed consent. Providers' special expertise—including knowledge of the changing nature of side effects and of the experiences of other users—can provide a sound basis for discussion. For example, a provider may conclude that a stated reason for removal is likely not directly linked to the device or that there may be ways to increase user satisfaction without changing methods. It is appropriate to share this information with the patient. Nonetheless, counselling should proceed with care and respect. Providers must inform patients that the purpose of the discussion is to support the patient and that the provider will remove the implant. Providers should not condition removals on what *they* consider "good reasons" provided by the patient.

6. Long-Term Contraceptives and Sexually Transmitted Diseases. *Pregnancy prevention and disease prevention are different goals. Providers should not use contraceptives as a lever to promote protection against STDs. This wrongly influences use.*

None of the available long-acting contraceptives provide protection against sexually transmitted disease. Indeed, that lack may be a source of confusion for users, who must take additional steps to protect against sexually transmitted diseases. Also, while the long-term methods retain their contraceptive effect, patients may fail to see health care providers, decreasing opportunities for regular sexually transmitted diseases screenings. Nonetheless, providers should not use contraceptives as a lever to promote protection against sexually transmitted diseasess. Pregnancy prevention and disease protection are different goals, and for a variety of complex reasons unknown to the health care provider, patients may not be equally motivated to take steps to achieve both. It is appropriate for providers to explain the risks of disease and to strongly urge a patient to take steps that enhance protection against sexually transmitted diseases, particularly patients at high risk. However, the final choice rests with the patient, and the patient should understand this.

7. Directive Counseling to Use Long-Acting Contraceptives.
Although health care providers ordinarily do not attempt to promote the use of any particular contraceptive method, in some cases directed counseling to consider using a long-term method is justifiable. Providers should develop and be guided by specific practice protocols that identify appropriate cases and require adherence to principles including informed consent, respect for each patient, and the avoidance of bias.

At a minimum, health care providers help patients make an informed decision about contraception by providing them with general information about contraceptive interventions and particularized information about their medical condition. However, contraceptive choice also rests on a complex of factors, including the patient's past experiences with contraceptives, her present life circumstances and relationships, her future goals and personal habits, and even unconscious motivations. Accordingly, providers ordinarily lack the competence to weigh the risks and benefits of different contraceptives for a patient and identify one as clearly superior. That judgment rests with the patient.

Nonetheless, in a narrow set of cases, providers will be justified in strongly urging a patient to try a highly effective long-acting method. Providers sometimes encounter a patient who has experienced a series of unintended, unwanted pregnancies based on a failure to prevent pregnancy successfully using other methods or a patient who is overwhelmed by the circumstances of her life and barely able to care for herself and her children. Perhaps she abuses alcohol or other drugs that impair her ability to use contraceptives or fulfill parental responsibilities and that would harm a developing fetus. She may be a sexually active teenager whose general level of maturity and known behaviors strongly indicate she is ill suited to manage the daily requirements of oral contraceptives or barrier methods.

In these kinds of circumstances, if a provider describes the range of contraceptive options and a patient has not decided to use a long-acting method, the provider is justified in urging her to try one. This rests on the provider's high degree of certainty regarding the individual's inability to avoid conception effectively by other available means and a high degree of certainty that under the circumstances unintended pregnancy will substantially harm the patient, her children, or future children. Arguably, a provider who forms a principled opinion of this kind yet fails to share it with the patient risks depriving her of beneficial information and support and neglecting obligations of care.

To help assure the responsible exercise of this influence, health care providers ought to articulate specific practice protocols to guide their conduct. For example, principles of informed consent must be honored and each patient treated with respect and dignity: strong recommendations become wrongful influences if they veer into bullying. The power differences that often exist between health care providers and patients heighten the risk of wrongful influence. Providers must also work to avoid biases. In counseling situations involving poor women and women who have otherwise been marginalized, there is a risk that providers will underestimate these women, overlooking the fact that they make even more complex life decisions in other contexts. The sensitive task of developing good protocols to guide this directive counseling will be aided by the participation of persons who have faced similar circumstances and who therefore may have important, unique insights to share.

8. Financial Barriers to Access. *It is appropriate for providers explicitly to address the high costs of an expensive contraceptive such as Norplant. Responses may include seeking financing for patients, covering cost considerations in informed consent discussions, and devising just ways to ration limited contraceptive supplies.*

For many women, the initial high cost of Norplant will prove a substantial barrier to access, despite the fact that its unique features may make it highly suitable for them.[19] Providers must determine how best to care for patients in the face of this financial obstacle. For example, providers with patients unable to pay for the method should consider exploring alternative financing arrangements such as loan funds, installment plans, or possible government or charitable financing rather than simply counselling patients to use less costly contraceptive alternatives. It is appropriate to include as part of informed consent discussions the risk that hundreds of dollars will be lost if the patient discontinues the method soon after it is initiated and that Norplant is unlike a less costly contraceptive in this respect.

Where limited government funds are involved, Norplant's expense can restrict the number of devices available to meet patient needs. When full funding is not available, it is appropriate for providers to identify ways justly to ration contraceptive supplies. For example, some providers may rely on waiting lists and a first-come, first-served approach. Others will try to identify patients unlikely to remain with the method after it is initiated and recommend that they try alternatives in light of clinical shortages. Providers may decide to tailor purchasing decisions to favor less expensive contraceptives in order to reach more patients. In all cases, providers should honestly and clearly communicate their fiscal constraints to patients. Over time, we should create mechanisms for allocating scarce health care resources in clinical settings— and in the broader health care system—that allow for more direct involvement of patients in the decision-making process and make it more sensitive to their perspectives, their priorities, and their voices.

Summary

Realizing the promise of long-acting contraceptives depends on continuing efforts to distinguish appropriate from inappropriate policies and practices. The current debates concerning Norplant and other long-term methods generally have based ethical judgment on too slender a reed. It is insufficient and overly divisive to limit the tools of analysis to questions of freedom and coercion. A richer perspective is needed. We have sketched out an alternative approach that rests on a close, case-by-case analysis attentive to the social dimensions and consequences of contraceptive decision making as well as to the individual interests at stake. The approach also takes special note of the need for access to long-acting contraceptives, the possibility for mistaken nonuse as well as mistaken use, and our country's past and present biases and power imbalances.

We do not claim that this method will make judgments about justifiable or unjustifiable influence easy or automatic. However, it should prove adept at underscoring the factors that require particular scrutiny. Perhaps more importantly, the approach highlights that influences for the use of long-acting contraceptives ought to be judged, not merely dismissed.

NOTES

1. See for example *People v. Johnson,* No. 29390 (Cal. Super. Ct. Tulare County 1990); *People v. Smith,* No. 92-CF-761 (Ill. Cir. Ct. McLean County 1993); *State v. Carlton,* No. CR90-1937 (Neb. County Ct. Lincoln County 1991).

2. Women's Legal Defense Fund, *Legislation and Litigation Involving Norplant* (Washington, D.C.: Women's Legal Defense Fund; June 1992): 1–5 [hereinafter WLDF 1992]; Women's Legal Defense Fund, *Norplant Legislation and Litigation— 1993*: 1–6 (Washington, D.C.: Women's Legal Defense Fund, forthcoming) [herein-

after WLDF 1993]; Stacey L. Arthur, "The Norplant Prescription: Birth Control, Woman Control, or Crime Control?" *UCLA Law Review* 40 (1992): 1–101; Julie Mertus and Simon Heller, "Norplant Meets the New Eugenicists: The Impermissibility of Coerced Contraception," *St. Louis University Public Law Review* 11 (1992): 359–83; Board of Trustees, American Medical Association, "Requirements or Incentives by Government for the Use of Long-Acting Contraceptives," *JAMA* 267 (1992): 1818–21.

3. "Baltimore's Lead in Contraception," *New York Times*, 14 December 1992, A16.

4. Philip R. Reilly, *The Surgical Solution: A History of Involuntary Sterilization in the United States* (Baltimore: Johns Hopkins University Press, 1991), 1–11; Janet F. Ginzberg, "Compulsory Contraception as a Condition of Probation: the Use and Abuse of Norplant," *Brooklyn Law Review* 58 (1992): 979–1019.

5. Jacqueline Darroch Forrest and Lisa Kaeser, "Questions of Balance: Issues Emerging from the Introduction of the Hormonal Implant," *Family Planning Perspectives* 25 (1993): 127–32; Jennifer J. Frost, "The Availability and Accessibility of the Contraceptive Implant from Family Planning Agencies in the United States, 1991–1992," *Family Planning Perspectives* 26 (1994): 4–10.

6. Employee Benefit Research Institute, "Health Benefits-Coverage," in *EBRI Databook on Employee Benefits* (Washington, D.C.: Employee Benefit Research Institute, 3rd ed. 1995): 235–288.

7. Lisa Kaeser, "Public Funding and Policies for Provision of the Contraceptive Implant, Fiscal Year 1992," *Family Planning Perspectives* 26 (1994): 11–16. This article documents the almost total absence of state policies extending Medicaid funding of Norplant removals to women who initiate the method while on Medicaid, but become ineligible for Medicaid while the method is in place.

8. Kaeser finds that in Oklahoma, Medicaid coverage is denied for Norplant removals prior to the end of its five-year period of effectiveness unless a "medical reason" is provided for removing the device.

9. Elise Jones and Jacqueline Durroch Forrest, "Teenage Pregnancy in Developed Countries: Determinants and Policy Implications," *Family Planning Perspectives* 17 (1985): 53–63; Planned Parenthood Federation of America, "Sexuality and Reproductive Behavior Among U.S. Teens," fact sheet, February 1991.

10. Margaret Polaneczky, Gayle Slap, Christine Forke, Aviva Rappaport, and Steven Sondheimer, "The Use of Levonorgesrel Implants (Norplant) for Contraception in Adolescent Mothers," *NEJM* 331 (1994): 1201–6.

11. Rebecca Maynard and Anu Rangarajan, "Contraceptive Use and Repeat Pregnancies Among Welfare-Dependent Teenage Mothers," *Family Planning Perspectives* 26 (1994): 198–205.

12. See note 5 above. Frost finds that nearly one-quarter of all family planning agencies surveyed had policies that condition minors' use of Norplant on parental consent.

13. Jason DeParle, "States' Eagerness to Experiment on Welfare Jars Administration," *New York Times*, 14 April 1994, A1, B10.

14. WLDF 1992, 1–5. WLDF 1993, 1–6.

15. Ginzberg, "Compulsory Contraception": 979–1019.

16. WLDF 1992, 1–5. WLDF 1993, 1–6.

17. Melissa Burke, "The Constitutionality of the Use of the Norplant Contraceptive Device as a Condition of Probation," *Hastings Constitutional Law Quarterly* 20 (1992): 207–46.

18. Mertus and Simon, "Norplant Meets the New Eugenicists": 359–83; John A. Robertson, *Children of Choice: Freedom and the New Reproductive Technologies* (Princeton, N.J.: Princeton University Press, 1994): 22–42, 69–93.

19. Frost, "The Availability and Accessibility of the Contraceptive Implant": 10.

PART II: Long-Acting Contraception in Context

KATHLEEN E. POWDERLY
Contraceptive Policy and Ethics: Lessons from American History

GEORGE F. BROWN
Long-Acting Contraceptives: Rationale, Current Development, and Ethical Implications

KATHLEEN E. POWDERLY

Contraceptive Policy and Ethics: Lessons from American History

It is often said that if we are unaware of our history, we are doomed to repeat the mistakes of the past. Many ethical and policy issues have been raised regarding long-acting contraceptives. While the technology of long-term contraceptives is relatively new, many of the dilemmas which occur are not. Mistakes and dilemmas regarding birth control are particularly apparent when the social historian looks at it from the perspectives of the women involved, rather than as a success of technology developed by the great men of medicine.

Advocates for birth control generally intended it to be an option for all women, regardless of race or class. The reality, however, was often that poor, otherwise unempowered women, often from minority groups, were most in need of such advocacy. Upper-class women had access to information and methods of birth control through their private physicians. They could pay for whatever was available. They voluntarily reduced the number of children they had. The well-intentioned efforts on the part of advocates for birth control to improve access for poor minority women often had the effect of targeting these women for efforts to reduce the numbers of children they had. The ability of a woman to choose the number of children she had and when she had them might have allowed her to control other aspects of her life and family and to improve the quality of life for herself and others. It could also come dangerously close, on a population level, to achieving the desires of eugenicists to reduce the numbers of poor minority people in the population.

The African-American community in Baltimore in the 1990s is concerned that offering Norplant to young African-American women who have already had a baby and are attempting to finish high school will result in a decrease in the number of African-American babies and is eugenic. Proponents believe that offering safe, effective, reversible, long-acting contraceptives will allow these young women to control their own destinies, finish school, and decide when and if they want more children. This tension is similar in many ways to that involving immigrant Irish and Eastern European women in the late nineteenth century. There was a real concern on the part of eugenicists that the immigrant population was growing and reproducing while educated, upper-class American women were successfully reducing the size of their families. Eugenicists may have wanted to control the fertility of immigrant women in order to maintain population proportions. On the other hand, early advocates for birth control might have wanted to improve access to birth control in order to empower these women to control their own destinies to a certain extent. Promoting the autonomy of women and acting beneficently on their behalf, in this case, comes dangerously close to the less ethically acceptable motivations of the eugenicists.

The history of the birth control movement in this country over the past 125 years provides clear examples of the tensions which have always existed between empowering women to control their fertility and promoting limitations on fertility for the disadvantaged. While the following is not an exhaustive history, several important developments in the history of the American birth control movement have been chosen to illustrate these tensions and provide a context within which to analyze contemporary policy dilemmas.

Contraception in Late Nineteenth Century America

Victorian beliefs regarding sexuality accepted promiscuity as a fact of life for men who were either not expected to or were unable to control their sexual urges. Women, on the other hand, were expected to control or even deny their sexuality.[1] Prostitutes were a common and accepted solution to this dichotomy. Despite the view that female sexuality was viewed as inextricably linked to reproduction, contraception was widely practiced among all social classes. The methods employed varied by class, however, due to cost and availability. The upper classes were more likely to use relatively expensive methods of contraception such as condoms, spermicides, and douches. They might also have had access to diaphragms and cervical caps which were smuggled in from Europe at a high cost. Withdrawal and rhythm were often the only methods available to the poor. In an era when menstrual cycles were poorly understood, pregnancies often resulted. Abortion, often self-induced and always dangerous, was resorted to frequently. It is estimated that one out of every five to six pregnancies in America ended with an abortion by the 1850s.[2] Mortality from septic abortions was extremely high. In 1888, it was estimated as being fifteen times greater than maternal mortality.[3]

During this era, American feminists supported the concept of "voluntary motherhood."[4] Far from empowering women and providing them with sexual freedom, however, voluntary motherhood sustained traditional family roles for women. Limitation of family size enhanced their ability to fulfill their societal roles as wives and mothers according to this view. The feminists were joined by moral reformers who were concerned about excessive breeding among the lower classes. Immigrants were particular targets of this concern. Focusing efforts toward reduction of fertility on the lower class and members of minority groups has strong historical roots in the late nineteenth century.

Although contraception was widely practiced in private and abortion accepted as a necessity when it failed, many were not willing to risk expressing support for them in public or admitting to their use. This reluctance influenced public policy. Abortion was declared illegal for the first time in the United States in 1830. A majority of states had declared it so by 1870.[5] A great legal blow was dealt to contraception in 1873 with the passage of the statute that came to be known as the Comstock law. This federal statute made it illegal to transport obscene materials through the mail. Contraceptive devices such as condoms and diaphragms as well as literature were confiscated under this law, which was in effect until 1936. It lost its power in a case in which Margaret Sanger established the right of doctors and other qualified professionals to use the mail for such distribution. Contraceptives themselves remained in the obscenity statutes until 1971.[6]

Margaret Sanger and the Movement for Planned Parenthood

Perhaps no name is more associated with birth control, family planning, and reproductive freedom for women than Margaret Sanger's. The daughter of Irish immigrants, Margaret was born in 1879 and played a strong role in the birth control movement in the United States and abroad until her death in 1966. While her decision to devote her life to the promotion of access to birth control for all women was influenced by many factors, her own family background certainly played an important role. Margaret was the middle child in a family of eleven. She was impressed at a young age with the effect of frequent pregnancies on her mother, who suffered from tuberculosis and died at the age of fifty. Her mother's frequent pregnancies and their ultimate role in her early death angered Margaret.

Margaret was trained as a nurse, although she left her training program early to marry William Sanger. Because of prohibitions against married nursing students in this era, she could not remain in the program. Her marriage produced three children. Margaret remained conflicted throughout her life between her obligations to her children and the demands of her cause—access to birth control for all women. This conflict, of course, is very familiar to working mothers today.

Margaret Sanger's experience as a visiting nurse and midwife on New York's Lower East Side provided the stimulus for her crusade. She often cited the case of Sadie Sachs, a twenty-eight-year-old Jewish immigrant and mother of three who was married to a truck driver named Jake. Unable to deal with another pregnancy and an additional child, Mrs. Sachs nearly died from a self-induced abortion. Margaret nursed her for weeks and listened to her pleas for reliable contraception. It is likely that Margaret offered her personal experiences with condoms and coitus interruptus, the common methods of the day. Mrs. Sachs knew another pregnancy would kill her. Her physician advised her to "tell Jake to sleep on the roof." If only these immigrant men could control their sexuality, there wouldn't be so many problems! Her physician had no better or more constructive advice to offer her. Three months later, Mrs. Sachs died of septicemia. Her husband was distraught and her children left motherless. Margaret Sanger called it "the dawn of a new day in my life . . . I knew I could not go back merely to keeping people alive. . . ."[7] She was determined to empower women to control their own fertility and, consequently, their own destinies.

Early in her crusade, Margaret Sanger used her connections to the Socialist Party to promote her cause. She published a column entitled "What Every Girl Should Know" in *The Call*, a New York Socialist daily, in 1912 and 1913. The columns elicited a range of responses and were ultimately challenged by Anthony Comstock. Early in 1913, one of the columns was entitled "What Every Girl Should Know—Nothing; by order of the U.S. Post Office" and was followed by a blank space. Several weeks later the censored column appeared.[8] Birth control was not to become a priority issue for the Socialists, however. It couldn't compete with suffrage and labor issues.[9] Margaret was disillusioned and disappointed that birth control was not viewed by her comrades as a priority issue for women.

In 1914, Margaret abandoned her own failing marriage and devoted herself to the development of *The Woman Rebel*, a magazine for working women which would cover issues of sexuality and contraception. She was indicted under the Comstock laws for sending the first issue of this magazine through the mail. While awaiting trial, she wrote *Family Limitation*, a practical pamphlet on birth control methods. The world was about to go to war, and Margaret's arrest and cause were not receiving as much publicity as she had hoped for. She decided to flee the country and her children and go to Europe until she could command more visibility. While she continued her research on contraceptive methods, her husband, still a supporter, went to jail for dispensing one of her pamphlets. Margaret came back to heightened publicity for her cause and the charges against her were ultimately dropped.[10]

Sanger began a cross-country speaking tour to promote the importance of knowledge for women regarding sexuality and birth control. While she promoted access to birth control for all women, she focused particularly on the poor. Upper-class women had some access to contraception from their private physicians. Poor women did not. Margaret believed that uncontrolled fertility and large families were inextricably linked to poverty. Her efforts to empower poor women, however, would be viewed by some as racist and by others as having eugenic propensities. While many eugenicists supported the idea of limiting population growth, particularly among those they viewed as undesirable (e.g., the poor, immigrant groups, those with mental problems), they were greatly troubled by the idea that the upper classes would use birth control and the lower classes would continue to breed. The tension between empowering poor women to control their fertility for their own best interest and limiting fertility among the poor and the underclass persists to this day as we have seen in the debate about long-acting contraceptives.

Margaret Sanger brought birth control directly to the poor women of Brooklyn on October 16, 1916, when she opened a free-standing clinic in Brownsville. Immigrant women from many cultures lined up with their baby carriages to learn how to prevent future pregnancies. In the few weeks the clinic was open, 464 women were provided with sex education and contraceptive information.[11] The clinic was raided by the New York City Vice Squad and Margaret and her sister, Ethel Byrne, the clinic's nurse, were jailed. The trial produced an important legal victory for birth control. The New York State Court of Appeals interpreted the law to allow for prescription of contraceptives by physicians not only to prevent or cure venereal disease—an interpretation largely applied to men—but also for any health reason. This opened the door for physicians to prescribe contraceptives for women. It also produced another dramatic effect, however. Birth control from that point on was a physician-dominated enterprise. While Margaret's Brownsville clinic brought contraception to the community level and to poor women, it did so at a price. Nurses, and to a large extent, women, were not to control the provision of contraceptives.[12] This is a legacy with which we live to this day. In populations with limited access to physicians, it is a clear disadvantage.

The compromises struck with the medical community are evident in Margaret Sanger's interactions with Robert Latou Dickinson. Dr. Dickinson, a Brooklyn gynecologist, was a champion of studies of female sexuality, fertility, and contraception. While he was not a strong supporter of contraception early in his career, he became one of its strongest supporters and was on the Board of Planned Parenthood at the time of his death in 1950 at the age of eighty-nine. Dickinson and Sanger both fought for the right to contraceptives, but he viewed her techniques as propagandist. He sought initially to evaluate the effectiveness of contraceptive counselling and techniques, using more traditional scientific methods. Influential in his field, Dickinson used his platform as president of the American Gynecological Society to promote professional interest in birth control. He set up a committee on maternal health at the prestigious New York Academy of Medicine to promote contraceptive research. He found, however, that without Margaret's "propaganda," he had trouble recruiting patients. While Dickinson had access to the medical establishment, Margaret had access to the women who would be the subjects of the research and the users of contraceptives. Dickinson also ultimately sought Margaret's assistance in securing diaphragms for his patients. He had been unable to acquire enough diaphragms through legal channels. Margaret had been smuggling them into the country, sometimes in Three-in-One oil boxes. She had married the millionaire head of the Three-in-One oil company and used his fortune and his facilities to promote her cause.[13] Sanger and Dickinson often disagreed vehemently on strategy, but also cooperated. Dickinson ultimately joined Margaret's Birth Control Clinical Research Bureau's advisory board. Together, they assured that birth control would be available to American women. It was, however, to be a male-dominated enterprise constructed on the medical model.

Sterilization

Tubal sterilization was first proposed in the early nineteenth century for effective long-term contraception in women undergoing Caesarean sections. It was not until the latter part of the century, however, when asepsis and safer anaesthesia were available, that it was attempted. The first reported tubal sterilization was performed by Samuel Lungren, an Ohio physician, in 1880.[14] While technology had evolved enough to attempt these procedures, it is important to recognize that they were still quite risky. A paper delivered at the Brooklyn Gynecological Society in 1891 reviewed the sixty-eight sections which had been performed in the U.S. from 1882–1891. The Brooklyn maternal mortality rate of 33 1/3% compared favorably with the national mortality rate of 40%.[15] Surely, if a woman survived one section, avoidance of another would be an important consideration. Many of the early tubal ligations were recommended for "protective" indications—i.e., to protect the life or health of the woman.[16]

After the turn of the century, however, eugenics was a dominant reason for tubal sterilization, particularly involuntary sterilization. Compulsory sterilization began to be recommended for individuals with hereditary disease, the "feeble-minded" (i.e., the insane and demented) and the mentally retarded. There were also racial overtones, as undesirable characteristics were perceived to occur more often in Negroes, Orientals, and the foreign-born. In addition, there were some moves to sterilize habitual criminals. While recommendations for habitual criminals dealt largely with men, efforts to control hereditary and mental illnesses were most often directed at women.[17] Efforts to train female inhabitants of mental institutions gave way to a priority to keep them from reproducing. The view that deviance was hereditary was supported in large part by studies of two families: the Jukes and the Kallikaks.

Richard Dugdale, a social reformer, studied 709 people over five generations in a family he called the "Jukes." Although Dugdale believed both heredity and environment were to blame for the propensity of the Jukes for crime, intemperance, and prostitution, he gave real credence to heredity.[18] He estimated that their care had cost society $1,308,000. In 1912, Henry Goddard added to the belief that deviance was hereditary with his publication of *The Kallikak Family*.[19] Goddard had been studying feeble-mindedness when he discovered the family, which he traced back over six generations. The progenitor had produced both a legitimate and an illegitimate line. The legitimate line produced upstanding citizens, while the illegitimate line produced large families with a disproportionate number of feeble-minded individuals.[20]

Already concerned with the effects of immigration on population demographics, eugenicists were given superb ammunition with these two studies. The eugenics movement also received financial support from some of the country's most prominent philanthropists, including Mrs. E. H. Harriman, John D. Rockefeller, Dr. John Harvey Kellogg, and Samuel Fels.[21] Even Theodore Roosevelt supported the movement, urging Americans to avoid "racial suicide"—the upper classes must not be outnumbered in their progeny by immigrants and the lower class.

The nation's first involuntary sterilization law was passed in 1907 in Indiana. California followed suit in 1909 and by 1913, fourteen states had laws allowing involuntary sterilization.[22] The effect of the laws varied. From 1907 to 1921 there were 3233 documented sterilizations performed under state laws. These sterilizations were seen by many within the mental hygiene movement as beneficial to society and, at the very least, as not harmful to the individual. On the other hand, seven of the laws were declared unconstitutional.[23] While there was much popular and professional support, eugenic sterilization was still controversial. Additional statutes drafted with more concern regarding constitutional constraints and more care about guardians' consent were more successful. Ultimately, the Supreme Court provided a boost for involuntary sterilization with its decision in *Buck v. Bell* in 1927.

Oliver Wendell Holmes wrote: "It is better for all the world, if instead of waiting to execute degenerative offspring for crime, or to let them starve for their imbecility, society can prevent those who are manifestly unfit from continuing their kind." The number of states with sterilization laws increased to thirty and the number of involuntary sterilizations increased dramatically.[24] Philip Reilly, a prominent researcher in this field, reaches the following conclusions: (1) that more than 60,000 persons were sterilized under state laws in thirty states; (2) that sterilization programs were active through the 1940s and 1950s and not influenced by reactions to Nazi sterilization programs; and (3) that there was a dramatic increase in the percentage of women who were sterilized after 1930.[25] Eugenic sterilization virtually disappeared after the 1960s in an era of awareness of patients' rights and, most especially, the need for society to protect the vulnerable. The major ethical conflict regarding sterilization today is balancing the rights of a mentally retarded or mentally disabled person to sexual freedom with a protection of their best interests regarding childbearing. Even in cases where it is clear that the individual has no ability to comprehend pregnancy and childbirth and may be harmed by the experience, it is difficult to obtain a court order for sterilization because of the history of abuses. Perhaps it is more beneficent to take the middle ground in these cases. While routine sterilization of a mentally impaired individual without her consent is clearly wrong, restricting the sexual expression of a profoundly impaired individual who cannot comprehend her sexuality, much less pregnancy or coitus-related contraception, is also not justified. In carefully considered circumstances, advocates for the patient may conclude that sterilization is in the patient's best interest. The prominence of this issue in the Senate confirmation hearings of Dr. Henry Foster illustrates the importance of this issue and the lack of societal consensus even today.

Ethical issues have also come up in voluntary sterilization of mentally competent individuals. Some women, particularly poor women, have not had access to desired sterilization. Married women were sometimes required to have their husband's consent or were denied sterilizations until they had produced a certain number of children. Young, nulliparous women were also not considered candidates for tubal sterilizations. While tubal ligations are sometimes successfully reversed, they should be considered as permanent when they are done. Parity, marital status, and age, while important factors for the woman to consider, should not be used to deny her a tubal sterilization if she really desires one. Sterilizations have sometimes been advocated for women with serious medical conditions such as tuberculosis, diabetes, or cardiovascular disease. While these may be important medical indications, it is important to recognize that they are conditions more common among the poor and women of color.[26] Thus what may appear to be a well-intentioned medical intervention may be perceived as racist or as promoting eugenics. Counselling regarding sterilization as a contraceptive option must be done with sensitivity to the historical context.

Birth Control and the Modern Era

The 1960s and 1970s saw great technological advances in contraception. The development and approval of oral contraceptives finally provided a highly effective form of contraception which was not associated with individual sexual acts. Intrauterine devices also became popular choices for women and couples who wanted to control fertility. Although IUDs would later become less available because of legal challenges related to side effects of the Dalkon Shield, they were a method of choice for many women during this time.

In addition to technological advances, there were legal and policy victories for birth control. A significant victory in this regard occurred in New York City in 1957 when Dr. Louis M. Hellman fitted a severely diabetic postpartum woman with a diaphragm in violation of the policies of the commissioner of hospitals. The media had been notified in advance and the resulting coverage precipitated a policy change which allowed women to receive contraceptive counselling and devices in municipal hospitals in New York City.[27] Dr. Hellman went on to serve as deputy assistant secretary for population affairs in the Department of Health, Education, and Welfare under President Nixon. He oversaw the Title X family planning initiatives which provided family planning services to five million women who desired them but could not afford them.

The Supreme Court declared contraception a constitutional right for married couples in 1965.[28] The Comstock laws were finally repealed in 1971 and the Supreme Court guaranteed a woman's right to abortion in *Roe v. Wade* in 1973.[29] Women were entitled to access to contraceptives and abortion services. This, however, did not ensure that they would have access. Some women did not have access to Title X funded services and could not afford contraceptives. Barriers to health care in general often extended to family planning services. For others, partners or spouses prohibited the use of desired contraceptives. In addition, the fight against legalized abortion rages on and has escalated to violent outbursts which threaten the providers and users of abortion services. There is also the danger that women who do not desire contraceptives will be coerced into using them by partners or social pressures.

Conclusion

There is an important historical context within which to view the current ethical and policy issues with long-acting contraceptives. Well-intentioned efforts to empower *all* women, including poor women of color, must be balanced with a keen sense of the abuses evident in the history of the birth control movement. Racism and eugenic concerns have been consistent issues in debates about controlling fertility, and our targeted educational programs and initiatives must be sensitive to community concerns. Empowering women to make their own reproductive choices is a praiseworthy goal. It can only be achieved if we maintain an awareness of the successes and failures in the history of the birth control movement.

NOTES

1. Linda Gordon, *Woman's Body, Woman's Right: Birth Control in America* (New York: Penguin, 1981).

2. Ellen Chesler, *Woman of Valor: Margaret Sanger and the Birth Control Movement in America* (New York: Simon & Schuster, 1992), 63.

3. M. A. La Sorte, "Nineteenth Century Family Planning Practices," *Journal of Psychohistory* 4 (1976): 163–83.

4. Linda Gordon, 95–115.

5. La Sorte, 163–83.

6. Dorothy Wardell, "Margaret Sanger: Birth Control's Successful Revolutionary," *American Journal of Public Health* 70, no.7 (1980): 736–42.

7. Chesler, 63; Wardell, 736–42; Margaret Sanger, *Margaret Sanger: An Autobiography* (New York: W.W. Norton, 1938), 89–92; Margaret Sanger, *My Fight for Birth Control* (New York: Farrar Rinehart, 1931), 46–65.

8. Chesler, 65–66; Sanger, *Autobiography*, 111.

9. Chesler, 97–99.

10. Chesler, 102–4, 140.

11. Chesler, 150.

12. Chesler, 159–60.

13. Wardell, 741.

14. S. S. Lungren, "A Case of Caesarean Section Twice Successfully Performed on the Same Patient," *American Journal of Obstetrics* 14 (1881): 78; A. M. Siegler and A. Grunebaum, "The 100th Anniversary of Tubal Sterilization," *Fertility and Sterility* 34 (1980): 610.

15. Minutes of the Brooklyn Gynecological Society, vol. 1, 1890–1899. Archives of the Medical Research Library of Brooklyn, SUNY Health Science Center, Brooklyn.

16. Per E. Bordahl, "Tubal Sterilization: A Historical Review," *The Journal of Reproductive Medicine* 30, no.1 (1985): 19.

17. Philip R. Reilly, *The Surgical Solution* (Baltimore: The Johns Hopkins University Press, 1991).

18. R. L. Dugdale, *The Jukes: A Study in Crime, Pauperism, Disease and Heredity* (New York: G.P. Putnam & Sons, 1877).

19. H. H. Goddard, *The Kallikak Family* (New York: Macmillan, 1912).

20. Reilly, *The Surgical Solution*, 20–22.

21. Philip Reilly, "Involuntary Sterilization in the United States: A Surgical Solution," *The Quarterly Review of Biology* 62, no. 2 (1987): 153–70.

22. Reilly, "Involuntary Sterilization," 154–55.

23. Reilly, "Involuntary Sterilization," 158.

24. Reilly, "Involuntary Sterilization," 160.

25. Reilly, "Involuntary Sterilization," 161.

26. Barron Lerner, "Constructing Medical Indications: The Sterilization of Women with Heart Disease or Tuberculosis, 1905–1935," *Journal of the History of Medicine and Allied Sciences* 49 (1994): 362–79.

27. Louis M. Hellman, "Family Planning Comes of Age," *American Journal of Obstetrics and Gynecology* 109, no.2 (1971): 214–24.

28. *Griswold v. Connecticut,* 381 U.S. 479 (1965).

29. *Roe v. Wade,* 410 U.S. 113 (1973); Louis M. Hellman, "A History and Reminiscence of the Office of the Deputy Assistant Secretary for Population Affairs, Department of Health, Education and Welfare, 1969–1977," *Bulletin of the History of Medicine* 56 (1982): 77–87.

George F. Brown

Long-Acting Contraceptives: Rationale, Current Development, and Ethical Implications

Long-acting contraceptive methods have played a prominent role in international family planning programs. The emphasis placed on these methods is linked to the demographic perspective that has motivated many of these programs. In this review, the rationale for long-acting contraceptives is examined along with the research and development process through publicly financed efforts. The current status of new methods under investigation is described, and the ethical implications of long-acting contraceptives are discussed. A careful analysis of the ethical dimensions of long-acting methods is needed to inform research and development strategies and especially the policies and procedures of family planning programs as they employ these methods.

The Rationale for Long-Acting Contraceptives

International concern about rapid population growth was the primary motivation for the establishment of national family planning programs, beginning with India in 1952. Anxiety about rapid population growth engendered great concern about reducing high fertility in developing countries and overshadowed the concern for the reproductive rights and health of individuals. In order to achieve high levels of continuous contraceptive practice, priority was attached to modern contraceptives, especially long-acting methods and sterilization. Methods requiring repeated actions by the user were given lower status in many countries on the grounds that they were too difficult for women and men to use consistently.[1]

The modern era of long-acting contraception began in the early 1960s, with the development of the first modern intrauterine device, the Lippes Loop. It closely followed the development and introduction of oral contraceptives. The impact of these two new contraceptive methods was enormous:

for the first time it seemed possible that modern contraceptive technology would enable women in poor countries to limit the size of their families.

As a result of this enthusiasm for modern technologies, user-controlled barrier methods, despite their important historical role in industrialized countries, were relegated to second-class status. Diaphragms were considered too difficult to fit or to use consistently and were given such low status that they became unavailable in many countries. Other barrier methods were made available, but were accorded lower priority. Family planning program managers and international agency officials championed the "cafeteria approach," offering a wide range of methods to women and men. But modern, long-acting methods including sterilization were emphasized, both in research and in service delivery.

While the oral contraceptive was quickly introduced and widely accepted by women in most industrialized countries, public health and family planning officials were skeptical about the ability of women in developing countries to use this technology effectively and continuously. The IUD, on the other hand, was greeted with great enthusiasm, because it didn't require any motivation or action on the part of women after insertion, and it would remain in place for many years.[2] Early experience in Taiwan was positive, and although problems with side-effects and spontaneous expulsion were recognized, the IUD was perceived as the prototype of the ideal contraceptive. By 1993, over sixty million Copper-T IUDs had been inserted worldwide.

Thus the search for improved long-acting contraceptives intensified. The pharmaceutical industry, however, showed little interest in long-acting methods or contraceptive development of any kind. The reasons for the decline of the pharmaceutical industry research and development are many and include: more stringent and costly testing requirements by the US Food and Drug Administration, longer time required for development which results in reducing the years of patent protection, negative publicity about new contraceptives, and increased product liability, among others.[3] Drug companies focussed mostly on making improvements in oral contraceptives and withdrew from research on new long-acting methods.

The research for improved contraceptives aimed for characteristics that seemed to have the greatest potential in developing countries with low levels of literacy. The "ideal" method would have the following characteristics:

- long-acting
- highly effective, as close to 100% as possible
- safe
- few or no side effects

- fully reversible
- application not coitus-related
- no need for continuing supplies
- little or no need for action on the part of the user after initial acceptance
- low cost.[4]

Such a contraceptive would, in all likelihood, require the actions of a trained health provider to initiate and to stop the use of the method. There was little discussion of the relative values of provider-dependent methods and user-controlled ones other than the requirements for training and sound medical technique that might be required of the former.

Ironically, another method, having virtually all the desired features save one, became increasingly widely used throughout the seventies and eighties. This method was sterilization. Despite its irreversibility, female sterilization became the most widely used method of contraception throughout the world. By 1993, over 170 million sterilizations had been performed. Male sterilization also grew in popularity, although at a lower rate.[5]

The search for new long-acting reversible contraceptives intensified. Ethical concerns about sterilization were greatly heightened by the coercive practices employed during the Indira Ghandi emergency period in India in the mid-seventies.[6] This experience, and the potential of coercive use of sterilization in other countries, further fueled the effort to find better long-acting methods that would be fully reversible.

With the strong support of U.S. foundations, and later of the United States, other western governments, and United Nations agencies, several public institutions initiated contraceptive research and development programs beginning in the early 1970s. Donor funding was primarily from international development assistance accounts which were focussed on the needs of developing country populations and only secondarily on the developed world's needs.

Unlike industry, the public sector contraceptive development programs are nonprofit, and are devoted primarily to designing, testing, and introducing methods that would be acceptable and easy for public health programs in the developing world to utilize. These public sector groups include: the World Health Organization, the Population Council, Family Health International, CONRAD (Contraceptive Research and Development Program), the National Institutes of Health and Human Development, and the South-to-South Program. Several developing countries, notably India, China, and Mexico, established significant contraceptive research and testing programs.

The underlying philosophy of the contraceptive development enterprise was that poor women in developing countries would have great difficulty using any method that required repeated application, that was coitus-related, or that required extensive education and training. But early experience in several Asian countries demonstrated that following initial acceptance, many women had low continuation rates, especially with oral contraceptives but also with IUDs. Low contraceptive continuation rates were seen to be a major obstacle to reducing fertility.[7] This suggested to researchers and donors that even greater priority needed to be given to the development of highly effective long-acting methods that would be more acceptable to users for extended periods.

The Contraceptive Development Process

The development of a new contraceptive typically takes ten to twenty years and can cost thirty million dollars or more, depending on the number of compounds that must be tested.[8] Modifications and improvements of existing methods can be quicker and cheaper. Public sector agencies must collaborate with private industry if new compounds are to be tested. Frequently, companies have compounds that might be candidates for research, but have not proceeded to investigate them. Public sector research groups must negotiate agreements with companies in order to obtain access to promising compounds. Typically, public sector price protection is negotiated at this point in order to minimize the cost that will ultimately be charged to not-for-profit family planning programs internationally.

Public sector development involves early testing of compounds in the laboratory, animal studies of effectiveness and toxicity, followed by small-scale studies on humans. These studies determine metabolic effects, contraceptive effectiveness, safety, and side effects of the method. Different dosage levels and formulations and sometimes comparative trials of different compounds are undertaken. If the compound appears to be safe, effective, and have few or no side effects, large-scale trials are conducted. Meanwhile, manufacturing processes are developed in partnership with private industry, since full-scale manufacture is usually undertaken by a pharmaceutical company. If these steps are successful, an application is made for approval with a regulatory agency such as the U.S. Food and Drug Administration.

The process is rarely if ever as smooth as this outline suggests. Frequent setbacks, reformulations, and abandonment of candidate compounds occur. A significant degree of collaboration with private industry is almost always required, necessitating complex negotiations and, frequently, contractual limitations placed upon pricing and distribution rights. Since public sector agencies usually receive relatively short-term funding, it is difficult to maintain the necessary financial support throughout the course of the lengthy development process. Heavy costs are required toward the latter part of the process, when large-scale trials are conducted and manufacturing investments are needed.

Following regulatory approval, the product is marketed. Again, this is often a shared undertaking, with the public sector agency responsible for introducing the product to governments and not-for-profit entities and private industry marketing to the commercial sector. As a result of the earlier agreements with industry, a two-tier price structure is often applied in order to establish a low price for public organizations.

Over the past ten years a carefully planned international effort has been made to facilitate the introduction of new contraceptive methods in developing countries. The introduction of the Norplant implants has served as a prototype for other methods.[9] A series of steps are undertaken with a government interested in the new product. The cost of the method and the potential niche it may fill are important considerations. The capacity of the public health system and the requirements of the method need to be carefully assessed. A provider-dependent method, for example, requires a clinic system of good quality and trained health care personnel. Pre-introductory trials may be conducted to determine local acceptability, train providers and counsellors, and provide information for regulatory approval. Acceptability and program research is undertaken, followed by the elaboration of an introduction plan appropriate to the needs of the country. This includes mobilization of the existing public health infrastructure, training, informational materials for users and providers, logistics and supply, management information systems, and evaluation. A constant management feedback system is needed to identify problems and devise solutions.

Despite careful planning for introduction of Norplant implants, unforeseen problems arose in several countries. One important lesson is that more emphasis must be given to thorough consultation with women's health advocacy groups and relevant community groups as well as with individual users. Ethical considerations need to be examined in a timely fashion. The experience with Norplant implant introduction internationally serves as a valuable model for the future introduction of other new contraceptive methods.[10]

Because the time required to develop new contraceptive technologies is usually ten to twenty years, the contraceptive methods that are now emerging from the research and development pipeline were initiated in the seventies and early eighties, when priority was given to long-acting, highly effective provider-dependent methods. Thus many of the methods that are likely to become available before the year 2000 fit this profile. The review that follows describes those long-acting methods that are nearing completion and that are reasonably likely to be introduced by the turn of this century or soon thereafter. In addition, it briefly describes the development of user-controlled methods. This review does not claim to be complete and focusses largely on public sector research efforts. It does not describe the prospects of possible compounds undergoing research by the pharmaceutical industry. The inherent uncertainty of contraceptive research renders any firm predictions impossible.

Intrauterine Devices

Over the past decade, a series of advanced copper-bearing IUDs have been developed and introduced. Currently the two most widely used are the Copper-T 380 IUD (marketed in the U.S. as Paragard) and the Multiload IUD. Both are long-acting, highly effective, and inexpensive. The duration of use of the Copper-T 380 was recently extended by the FDA to ten years. These newer IUDs have a smaller risk of causing pelvic inflammatory disease. This risk is further decreased by careful selection of potential users. These devices should be limited to women who are in long-term monogamous relationships and who do not have a recent history of pelvic inflammatory disease.

Progestin-releasing IUDs are now ready for introduction. These IUDs release constant low doses of levonorgestrel, the same progestin that is used in Norplant implants and some oral contraceptives. They are extremely effective over a five-year period and may cause a smaller amount of blood loss than the copper-bearing IUDs, an especially important factor for anemic women. Cramping, pain, and risk of pelvic inflammatory disease may also be slightly reduced, but more data are needed to determine these differences. These devices are, however, more expensive than copper-bearing IUDs.

The likelihood of substantial new developments in IUD technology is not great, although new shapes and configurations of devices are being studied.[11]

Implant Systems

The successful development and introduction of Norplant implants has paved the way for a second generation of contraceptive implant systems. Norplant II, a two-rod implant, is undergoing large-scale clinical testing, and submission to the U.S. Food and Drug Administration was made in 1995. It is highly likely, therefore, that this method will be available for general use before the end of the decade. This implant should be equally as effective as the existing Norplant system and should have a duration of use of three to five years. Its advantage is greater ease of insertion and removal. In addition, since each implant is a solid rod rather than a capsule containing progestin crystals, it will be easier to manufacture.

A single implant system releasing the progestin nesterone is under investigation. This contraceptive would be especially appropriate for lactating women, since the progestin is not absorbed orally. Even if some of the hormone is found in the mother's milk, it will not be absorbed by the nursing infant. Two other single implant systems are under investigation, each using different progestins. The duration of use of these methods is likely to be significantly shorter than the Norplant system. Whether the obvious advantages of a single implant can be matched by other important qualities, including a significant duration of action, high levels of effectiveness, and low side effects, remains to be seen. It seems likely that at least one of these implant systems will reach the market by the end of this decade.

Biodegradable implants for women have been under study for a number of years. The potential advantage of eliminating the need for removal is offset by the fact that, after a certain period of time following insertion, the implant cannot be removed if the user desires. Thus far, research efforts have not been successful in moving this approach forward, and it is not possible to predict when or whether a biodegradable method will become available.

A two-implant system for men is undergoing development by the Population Council. One implant releases an analogue of a hypothalamic hormone to suppress sperm production, while the second releases an androgen to maintain normal sexual function. Both implants are currently expected to have a duration of one year. While early research results are encouraging, this method will not be available before the turn of the century, and it is not possible to predict when or whether it will be introduced.[12]

Injectables
The FDA approval in 1993 of Depo-Provera, a three-month injectable containing a progestin, represents the culmination of a long debate over this drug. It has been used in many countries for over twenty years, but approval in the U.S. was held back because of animal toxicity questions. This compound is highly effective and appears to be safe in long-term studies. A number of other injectable preparations using different progestins have been on the market internationally, although not in the United States. Noristerat is a progestin-only two-month injection which has been marketed internationally for several years. A monthly injectable, Cyclofem, was recently introduced by the World Health Organization. It is a combined progestin-estrogen compound. Like Norplant, progestin-only injectables produce menstrual irregularities. As Cyclofem combines estrogen and progestin, it mimics the normal menstrual

cycle. Since an injection cannot be reversed: any effects continue until the drug has worn off. Long-term effects of these injectable compounds are still under investigation, but no significant problems have been identified thus far.

New injectable formulations are under investigation in the hope of reducing side effects and increasing duration of action, but these goals have proven elusive thus far. Overall, a renewed interest in injectable contraception has followed the FDA approval of Depo-Provera in 1993. It is unlikely that any further significant advances will occur in this decade, but worldwide introduction efforts will likely enable existing methods to become more widely available.[13]

Vaccines

Contraceptive vaccines for women have been under investigation for two decades. Assuming that a safe and effective vaccine can be developed, the anticipated advantages would be ease of administration, convenience, the absence of any changes in the menstrual cycle, and low cost. Progress has been slow because of problems in developing the antigens needed to produce an immune response as well as difficulty in achieving a medium- or long-term fertility effect, among others. The most extensively studied approaches have used antibodies to human chorionic gonadotrophin, a hormone essential for the implantation and development of the embryo. Currently, a vaccine of this type might have a six- to twelve-month duration. New approaches using recombinant DNA technology have expanded the range of possibilities for vaccine research. Even when promising candidate antigens are identified, appropriate delivery systems need to be developed and tested. Another significant problem is the variability of the immune response among individuals. This means that the period of return to fertility will likely be unpredictable unless methods can be designed to neutralize the antibodies causing immunity. Given the complexity of this field of research, it is unlikely that a vaccine will reach the market in the next decade.

A male vaccine is also under investigation, based on an antigen to the hypothalamic hormone luteinizing hormone releasing hormone. Small-scale trials in humans have begun. A male vaccine would be especially interesting since no long-acting reversible method for men currently exists.[14]

Other Contraceptive Development Research

In addition to the research on long-acting methods described above, a number of other compounds are under investigation. The development of the antiprogestin drug mifepristone (RU 486) has been perhaps the greatest breakthrough in fertility control technology since the discovery of oral contraceptives. This drug and other analogues act by blocking the physiological effects of progesterone, which is essential to the maintenance of the embryo after implantation in the uterine lining. When used in sequence with a prostaglandin during early pregnancy, it is over 95% effective. It has been proven to be a safe and effective alternative to surgical abortion. Currently mifepristone is available in three European countries and in China. Political opposition has slowed the introduction and further testing of this method and has inhibited research on other analogues and on its use for other purposes. This could include once-a-month use, induction of missed menses, or as a post-coital emergency contraceptive. Research on analogue compounds and on alternative uses of mifepristone offer great potential for future advances in fertility regulation.[15]

Barrier methods for women and men have recently received significant renewal of interest. A re-examination of older methods, including the diaphragm and various spermicidal preparations, is under way. Two new products have recently been introduced: the vaginal sponge and the female condom. Although these methods offer women a greater choice for user-controlled contraception, each has limitations in effectiveness, acceptability, and a relatively high cost. A plastic condom for men is in an advanced state of development. It appears to have the advantage of long shelf-life and greater strength than latex condoms. It would also be resistant to petroleum-based lubricants, a limitation with latex condoms. New vaginal spermicidal compounds are being assessed against the standard used in most preparations, nonoxynol-9. A spermicide-releasing diaphragm is being tested, along with other barrier methods. An older method, a dissolvable film impregnated with spermicide, is being re-examined. If effective, it has the advantage of being simple to apply and is less messy than other vaginal applications.[16]

Contraceptive vaginal rings releasing low doses of hormones have been under investigation for over two decades. This approach has the benefit of being in the full control of the user, since, unlike the diaphragm, no special fitting is required. The woman can easily remove and reinsert the ring at any time. Several approaches have been studied, including a combined estrogen-progestin ring and a progestin-only formulation. Constant slow release of the hormone(s) results in absorption through the vaginal mucosa. The combination rings are used on a three-week-in, one-week-out schedule, while the progestin-only ring can be left in place for several months and removed at any time for cleaning. A ring containing the natural hormone progesterone has also been developed for use by lactating women. Side effects, including vaginal irritation, have slowed development. It seems likely, however, that at least one version of the vaginal ring will reach the market by early in the next century.[17]

The heightened concern about sexually transmitted diseases, especially HIV/AIDS, has resulted in a significant new effort to develop one or more vaginal microbicides that would block the transmission of the various microorganisms that cause sexually transmitted diseases. Ideally, at least two microbicides should be developed: one that would also prevent pregnancy and another that had no effect on fertility. The ideal method would have no side effects such as irritation of the vaginal mucosa, would be easy to apply, would not be messy, and would not be detectable by the male partner. A major research program has been initiated by the Population Council and other organizations to develop such products. Initial efforts are focussed on a group of coating agents called sulphated polysaccharides, which do not have a detergent effect, as do existing compounds.[18] Because microbicide research is in its early stages, it is impossible to predict how soon new methods will become available, but it is unlikely that this will occur before the end of the decade.

The lactational amenorrhoea method (LAM) and periodic abstinence have received attention by the World Health Organization, especially in identifying new methods to identify the fertile period. Male and female sterilization has benefitted by improved and simplified surgical techniques, and chemical agents to close the fallopian tubes are under investigation.

Ethical Considerations

Although reproductive rights have been among the rationales for family planning for many years, the rights of women to determine their child-bearing and to freely choose among contraceptive methods steadily became more strongly expressed throughout the 1980s. Women's health advocacy groups expressed deep concern about the demographic underpinnings of family planning programs in developing countries, which frequently downplayed women's reproductive rights in favor of state population policy.[19] Family planning researchers have stressed the need to improve the quality of family planning services, including the broader choice of methods.[20] Health problems associated with oral contraceptives and IUDs (especially the Dalkon Shield fiasco) became widely known. Overemphasis on targets and incentives for contraceptive acceptance in several developing countries resulted in instances of heavy-handed and coercive programs. In the United States, concerns have been expressed about programs targeted at poor and minority women. The introduction of the Norplant implant deepened this concern because of its dependence on health providers for insertion and removal and because of the efforts of some judges and legislators in the United States to try to use the Norplant method as a means to resolve legal and social problems.

Among other concerns has been the lack of attention given to the development of user-controlled methods. Suspicion of medical control over reproductive needs of women and the perceived dangers of hormonal methods and IUDs have been the key ethical issues that fueled the argument for the need to develop improved methods that can be utilized by women with no need for medical intervention.

The AIDS pandemic became widely recognized in the mid-1980s, and with it came a recognition that other sexually transmitted diseases had been almost totally neglected. As the only available methods of prevention were (and are) education about safer sex practices and the use of the condom, public health officials and women's health groups have realized that research priorities need to be changed. The limitations of the condom have become clearly evident: women cannot control condom use by their partners, and even raising the question can be dangerous in many situations.[21] Men frequently use condoms in extramarital relationships, but not at home. Thus women who are themselves monogamous and in long-term relationships can nonetheless be exposed to AIDS and other sexually transmitted diseases.[22]

In recent years, public health officials and women's health advocacy groups have emphasized the need for methods under the full control of women which can prevent the transmission of HIV and other sexually transmitted diseases as well as prevent pregnancy. In addition, research on new contraceptive methods for men is also receiving higher priority. At a recent international symposium of contraceptive research scientists, family planning program managers, and women's health advocates, recommendations called for these three objectives to receive high priority in future research.[23] Public sector agencies are already shifting their priorities to some degree to respond to these expressed needs.

Until recently, ethical issues have received insufficient attention in the context of new contraceptive development. The misuse of existing contraceptives, notably sterilization, has a long history. More recently, concerns about the use of Norplant implants in certain situations has attracted the attention of jurists, legislators, women's health advocacy groups, and ethicists. How can these concerns be incorporated into the process of selecting research priorities and avoiding potential ethical problems in the future?

It is important to remember that there are no intrinsic properties of contraceptives that have ethical limitations, provided that they are safe and are dispensed by competent providers and that users are fully counselled and choose voluntarily to adapt a method. The key issue is whether the family planning program and the individual provider of contraceptive information and services can ensure that the methods are offered in an ethically correct manner. The onus should be on the provider and the organization rather than on the method itself.

Nonetheless, provider-dependent long-acting contraceptives are more susceptible to ethical abuse than those that are user controlled. This is especially true of sterilization, which is a largely irreversible method, and of IUDs and implants, which necessitate insertion as well as removal by a provider.

Since a number of new implants and other provider-dependent methods will likely become available in the next decade, comprehensive measures need to be taken to ensure that ethical concerns are examined and addressed before and during the introduction of any new long-acting method. These concerns will have general application, but local conditions will play an important part in ethically sensitive introduction of new methods. For example, any provider-dependent method will require an adequate number of well-trained and skilled health practitioners and a minimum level of quality in clinical facilities and in client counselling. Removal necessitates an effective follow-up system. If these requirements cannot be met, the methods should not be introduced.

In areas where reproductive tract infections and sexually transmitted diseases are high, there is a need for combined use of condoms with long-acting methods. Providers in many countries are insufficiently attentive to the expressed needs and concerns of their clients. If users are not fully informed, do not have a fully voluntary choice of method, and cannot have easy access to removal or the ability to switch to another method, then any contraceptive technology may be used in an unethical fashion.

The capacity of the family planning and health delivery system in each country is a key factor in determining the appropriate use of different contraceptive methods. If the program has a weak medical and clinical infrastructure, provider-dependent methods should be limited or not used at all. The spread of such methods beyond the limited network of clinical facilities can present significant problems.[24] But arbitrarily limiting the use of such methods to countries with highly developed clinical systems presents problems as well. Most countries, for example, can use provider-dependent methods in urban hospitals. In each country an analysis of clinical capacity, the level of qualified providers, user preferences, and other factors needs to be made to determine the most appropriate mix of contraceptive methods to be included in a comprehensive family planning program.

At the level of the state, there may be a tendency to seek solutions to difficult social problems by promoting or even requiring the use of long-acting contraceptives that the user cannot easily reverse without medical intervention. It is essential to publicly debate what conditions are proper for use of a provider-dependent method in any given country or service setting. The

Norplant implant controversy in the United States has had the positive effect of elevating the debate publicly, and this should have a salutary impact on the introduction of future long-acting technologies as they emerge.

Other potential new methods, including vaccines and injectables, will each have their own ethical considerations. Special concern has been expressed by some groups concerning the potential inappropriate or abusive application of vaccines.[25] Since injections of all kinds are so widely used, vaccines for women or men could, for example, be given without the full knowledge or consent of the recipient. The fact that vaccines for women will have no effect on the menstrual cycle is an important advantage, but it can also enhance their potential for abuse since they will have no obvious side effects. Possible uncertainty about the individual variation in the time required to return to fertility also presents an ethical challenge if some women experience long periods of undesired infertility. Another concern is the potential confusion between contraceptive vaccines and other kinds of injections such as disease prevention vaccines. Thus an orally administered vaccine might be more desirable, since it would avoid such confusion. If a vaccine is developed, special care and ethical debate will be needed as it is considered for use in different country settings.

The cost of long-acting methods can have an ethical dimension. If the method is expensive, providers may be reluctant to remove it at the woman's request.

For all long-acting methods, the possibility of long-term health risks needs to be assessed. Even with the extensive research leading up to regulatory approval, it is not possible to ascertain with absolute certainty whether there might be rare long-term health problems once a method is introduced on a large scale. Post-marketing surveillance studies are therefore an essential requirement for new technologies. Such studies are under way with Norplant implants.

Obviously, user-controlled methods do not pose ethical issues as significant as provider-dependent contraceptives do. One ethical issue, however, is the availability of safe abortion services, since the failure rate is usually higher with user-controlled methods. Should such methods be encouraged in the absence of safe abortion services for contraceptive failure?

As for the contraceptive development community, there is a great need for closer interaction among scientists, women's health advocacy groups, consumer groups, ethicists, and users in order to shape research strategies. This is already happening in a systematic fashion,[26] and the expectation is that new contraceptive research will move even more vigorously in the direction desired by many women's health advocacy groups and others: the development of user-controlled methods and microbicides for women and contraceptives for men, with careful attention to ethical concerns.

Conclusion

It is likely that by the end of this century and early in the next, a small number of new long-acting contraceptives as well as a few new user-controlled methods will become available internationally. Not all will become available in the United States, however. Norplant II implants will almost certainly be introduced, and it is likely that a single implant will be marketed with other implant systems coming further in the future. A progestin-releasing IUD has been developed and will be introduced in several countries. A medical abortifacient, mifepristone, may be introduced in the United States and other countries by the end of the century. One or more barrier methods such as a new vaginal microbicide may also be developed.

It is much harder to predict the likelihood of new products emerging beyond ten to fifteen years, but a significant number of possibilities exist: vaccines for men and/or women, antiprogestins for once-a-month or menses-inducing purposes, new long-acting injectables, and an implant system for men, among others.

Many of the possible new methods are long-acting provider-dependent contraceptives. In large part this is a result of the research strategies established in the 1960s and 1970s, when priority was given to the development of highly effective long-acting contraceptives. Since the mid-1980s there has been a gradual shift in priorities toward the development of user-controlled methods, especially for women. Microbicides for women, male contraceptives, and post-coital methods are also important new priorities.

A further essential new priority should be to incorporate ethical considerations into all stages of contraceptive development and introduction. This must include ethical debate at the country level in order to inform legislative bodies, public health officials, and service providers as they seek to introduce new contraceptive technologies. The goal must be to expand the contraceptive choices of women and men by making available a range of methods in a voluntary, ethically responsible manner.

NOTES

1. George F. Brown, "Family Planning Programs," in *Technology in Society*, ed. George Zeidenstein (New York: Pergamon Press, 1987), 465–80; Judith Bruce and S. Bruce Schearer, "Contraceptives and Common Sense: Conventional Methods Reconsidered," *Population Council Public Issues Paper* (New York: Population Council, 1979), 1–101.

2. S. J. Segal, A. L. Southam, and K. D. Schafer, eds., *Intrauterine Contraception: Proceedings of the Second International Conference* (New York: Excerpta Medica Foundation, 1964), 9–13, 23–27.

3. Luigi Mastroianni, Jr., Peter Donaldson, and Thomas T. Kane, eds., *Developing New Contraceptives: Obstacles and Opportunities* (Washington: National Academy Press, 1990), 147–153; C. Wayne Bardin, "Public Sector Contraceptive Development: History, Problems, and Prospects for the Future," in *Technology in Society*, ed. George Zeidenstein (New York: Pergamon Press, 1987), 289–306.

4. Bernard Berelson, "Application of Intra-uterine Contraception in Family Planning Programs," in *Intra-uterine Contraception* (New York: Excerpta Medica Foundation, 1964), 9–13.

5. Amy E. Pollock, "One Hundred and Seventy Million Sterilizations Later: What We Know and What We Wish to Know," in *Contraceptive Research and Development 1984–94: The Road from Mexico City to Cairo and Beyond*, eds. P.F.A. Van Look and G. Perez-Palacios (New Delhi: Oxford University Press, 1994), 215–230.

6. D. R. Gwatkin, "Political Will and Family Planning: the Implications of India's Emergency Experience," *Population and Development Review* 5, no. 1 (1979): 29–59.

7. Bernard Berelson, "Demographic Requirements of Fertility Control Technology," PIACT Paper No. 1, Program for the Introduction and Adaptation of Contraceptive Technology (Seattle: 1978), 2–18 (available from PATH/PIACT, 4 Nickerson Street, Seattle, WA).

8. Bardin, "Public Sector Contraceptive Development," 292.

9. Joanne Spicehandler, "Norplant Introduction: A Management Perspective," in *Demographic and Programmatic Consequence of Contraceptive Innovations*, ed. S. J. Segal, A. O. Tsui, and S. M. Rogers (New York: Plenum Press, 1989), 199–223; K. J. Beattie, G. F. Brown, and M. M. Brady, "Expanding Contraceptive Choice: the Norplant Experience," in *Contraceptive Research and Development, 1984–1994*, 263–276.

10. Beattie, *Contraceptive Research and Development, 1984–1994*, 263–276

11. I. Sivin, "IUDs: A Look to the Future," in *Contraceptive Research and Development, 1984–1994*, 37–58.

12. R. Thau and A. Robbins, "New Implant Systems for Men and Women," in *Contraceptive Research and Development, 1984–1994*, 91–106.

13. J. Garza-Florez, M. C. Cravioto, and G. Perez-Palacios, "Contraceptive Research and Development: Injectables," in *Contraceptive Research and Development, 1984–1994*, 53–68.

14. N. J. Alexander, "Contraceptive Vaccines," in *Contraceptive Research and Development, 1984–1994*, 203–213; G. L. Ada and P. D. Griffin, eds., *Vaccines for*

Fertility Regulation (Cambridge: Cambridge University Press, 1991), p1 et seq. (the whole volume).

15. P. F. A. Van Look and H. Von Hartzen, "Post-Ovulatory Methods: The Emergence of Antiprogestins," in *Contraceptive Research and Development, 1984–1994,* 151–201.

16. L. J. D. Zaneveld, "Vaginal Contraception: Chemical and Physical Barriers," in *Contraceptive Research and Development, 1984–1994,* 69–90.

17. R. B. Thau and T. Jackanicz, "Contraceptive Vaginal Rings: A User-Controlled Long-Acting Method for Family Planning," in *Contraceptive Research and Development, 1984–1994,* 107–120.

18. C. J. Elias and L. L. Heise, "Challenges for the Development of Female-Controlled Vaginal Microbicides," *AIDS* 8 (1994): 1–9.

19. A. Germain, S. Nourojae, and H. H. Pyne, "Setting a New Agenda: Sexual and Reproductive Health and Rights," in *Population Policies Reconsidered*, ed. G. Sun, A. Germain, and L. C. Chen (Cambridge: Harvard University Press), 27–46.

20. Judith Bruce, "Fundamental Elements of the Quality of Care: A Simple Framework," *Studies in Family Planning* 21, no. 2 (1990): 61–91.

21. Dooley Worth, "Sexual Decision-Making and AIDS: Why Condom Promotion Among Vulnerable Women is Likely to Fail," *Studies in Family Planning* 20, no. 6 (1989): 297–307.

22. Christopher J. Elias and Lori L. Heise, "The Development of Microbicides: A New Method of HIV Prevention for Women," *Programs Division Working Paper*, no. 6 (New York: Population Council, 1993), 1–82.

23. Declaration of the International Symposium, "Contraceptive Research and Development for the Year 2000 and Beyond," in *Contraceptive Research and Development 1984–1994,* 543–546.

24. Karen Beattie and George F. Brown, "Expanding Contraceptive Choice: The Norplant Experience," in *Contraceptive Research and Development 1984–1994,* 263–276.

25. World Health Organization, *Fertility Regulating Vaccines* (Geneva: World Health Organization, 1993), 25.

26. World Health Organization, *Creating Common Ground* (Geneva: World Health Organization, 1994), 5–42. World Health Organization, *Creating Common Ground in Asia* (Geneva: World Health Organization, 1994), 5–38.

PART III: Exploring Conceptual and Theoretical Frameworks

BONNIE STEINBOCK

The Concept of Coercion and Long-Term Contraceptives

The ability to control one's fertility has long been recognized to be essential to women's equality and self-determination.[1] In some parts of the world, where death from childbirth or unsafe abortions is relatively common, it is a vital matter of health as well. Yet the choices available in contraception have been limited and most methods have disadvantages. The newest long-acting contraceptive on the scene, and the one that has received the greatest attention, is Norplant. After it was approved for use in the United States in December 1990, Norplant was widely hailed as a breakthrough, a nearly ideal contraceptive: safe, effective, easy to use. Yet Norplant has created bitter controversy. Precisely those features that help make it a nearly ideal contraceptive (its effectiveness and the fact that it works without women having to think about it) make it ideal for mandated contraception. Since Norplant is implanted on the inside of the upper arm, where it can be felt, and since it cannot be safely removed except by a trained practitioner, its continued usage can be monitored. This being the case, it is hardly surprising that within a few weeks of its approval by the FDA, an editorial in the *Philadelphia Inquirer* suggested that Norplant could be a useful tool for "reducing the underclass" by offering welfare mothers incentives to use Norplant. (The paper later apologized for the editorial and its racist overtones after protests from people inside and outside the paper.) Norplant's originator, Sheldon Segal, expressed outrage that a device intended to enhance reproductive freedom might be used coercively to restrict it.

Similar concerns about coercion were soon raised when bills were introduced in Kansas, Louisiana, Mississippi, Tennessee, and Ohio offering incentives to women on public assistance for using Norplant. Bills were also introduced in Kansas, Ohio, South Carolina, and Washington, all generally providing for the involuntary implantation of Norplant in substance-abusing women who had given, or might give, birth to drug-addicted children.[2] Most of these bills died in committee; a few are still pending.[3] The most famous court case involving Norplant occurred in Tulare County, California in January

1991, when Superior Court Judge Howard Broadman ordered Darlene John-son, who was convicted of child abuse, to use Norplant for three years as a condition of her probation. In April 1991, a trial judge in Indiana ordered a defendant to use Norplant after she allowed her boyfriend to kill her six-month-old son. Since 1966, there have been at least twenty cases in which judges have ordered criminal defendants to be sterilized, to practice contracep-tion, or to refrain from becoming pregnant.

A number of commentators view such legislation and court orders as examples of an assault on reproductive rights. They see parallels between past occurrences of sterilization abuse and the potential for coercive uses of Nor-plant. As an article in the *New York Times* expressed it:

> . . . the same qualities that make Norplant a boon to women may be a two-edged sword: some public health groups and women's advocates worry that the contraceptive could easily become an instrument of social control, forced on poor women and others whose fertility is seen as more of a threat to society than a blessing.[4]

Incentives aimed at women on public assistance, such as those proposed in Louisiana and Kansas, have been characterized as "clearly coercive, discrimi-natory, and a violation of those women's reproductive rights."[5]

However, it is often far from clear whether a given policy or program is coercive because the concept is complex, controversial, and often difficult to apply. For example, should we understand coercion narrowly, as involving only physical threats or force? Or can the offering of benefits and incentives to get people to do things they would otherwise not do be coercive? Intuitions differ as to whether a proposal *expands* or *constricts* a person's options, and so enhances or limits freedom. Moreover, the essentially normative nature of coercion claims entails that judgments about whether a policy is coercive embody substantive moral arguments about which reasonable people can dis-agree.

Despite the problematic nature of many coercion claims, the concept of coercion can be useful in evaluating social policies if the concept is carefully and appropriately used. To label a policy "coercive" is to make a *prima facie* objection to it. However, it should be remembered that coercion is not always unjustified or improper: for example, the coercive sanctions attached to the law to force individuals to obey it. Moreover, some socially desirable ends can only be achieved through mutually agreed-upon coercive policies, such as taxation and immunization.[6] Another problem is that too often coercion is used as a generalized term of abuse, without sufficient attention paid to the identifiable dimensions of the concept. Such intellectual sloppiness has two unfortunate results. First, it undercuts the charge of coercion where this is an apt and important moral criticism. Second, the overuse of coercion as a criticism creates the impression that there are no other reasons for objecting to social policies. Even if a policy is not correctly characterized as coercive, there may be other, equally important, objections to it. Incentives for birth control, for example, might be criticized as violating autonomy, equal protection, or informed consent, even if offering such incentives is not coercive.

After analyzing the concept of coercion in the first part of the paper, I apply the analysis in the second part to a range of cases: (1) mandated birth control for probationers; (2) financial incentives for women on public assistance; (3) the Dollar-a-Day program to prevent teenage pregnancy; and (4) Norplant in the Paquin School in Baltimore. The charge of coercion was leveled in all four situations but, I will argue, is plausible only in the first two.

The Concept of Coercion

Coercion, Voluntariness, and Responsibility

Coercion plays an important role in morality and the law because coercion typically acts as a *disclaimer of responsibility*. It has this role because coercion deprives people of free choice and thus makes what they do, to some extent, nonvoluntary.

The most clear-cut examples of coercion involve physical force or constraint. In the paradigm coercion situation, A says to B, brandishing a pistol, "Your money or your life." In what sense is B not acting according to his own free will? It is not that A deprives B of volition, as when A gets B to sign a contract by physically moving his hand, or by hypnotizing B. When B gives A his money, he does so deliberately and intentionally. He does what he most wants to do, given the situation. The coercion in this example is not the absence of volition, but rather *constrained volition*. Although intentional and deliberate, B's action is not done freely or autonomously.

The mere existence of external pressure or influence does not establish coercion. The influence or pressure exerted must be of a kind and amount that diminishes free choice. The central question for understanding the concept of coercion, then, is *how much, and what kind of, influence or pressure deprives actions and decisions of their autonomous character*. As we will see, the question does not have a simple or straightforward answer. Moreover, pressure or influence that does not qualify as coercive may also be morally objectionable if, for example, it exploits a person's desperate situation.

While the highwayman example is a clear case of coercion, we need a general theory of coercion to help us decide more controversial cases. Such a theory is given by Alan Wertheimer in his book, *Coercion*.[7]

Wertheimer's Two-Pronged Theory

This theory consists of two independent tests for coercion or duress, each of which is necessary and which are together jointly sufficient. The two prongs are:

1. The choice prong. A's proposal is coercive only if B has *no reasonable alternative but to succumb* to A's proposal.

2. The proposal prong. A's proposal is coercive only if it is *wrongful* (and not simply because it deprives B of free will and judgment). In general, if A has a right to do what he proposes, then his proposal is not wrongful (although it may be morally objectionable on other grounds).

Coercion as Normative

Note that the two-pronged theory is a moralized theory. That is, its conditions of application contain an ineluctable reference to moral rightness and wrongness. We cannot decide whether a proposal is coercive without talking about what A and B have a right to do or should do. Although a few philosophers have attempted to give morally neutral analyses of coercion,[8] there appears to be general agreement that the concept of coercion is inescapably normative.[9] To take a recent example from the law, a woman was convicted of homicide after she participated in the kidnapping of an executive who died. She claimed to be a battered wife and said that she was forced by her husband to participate. The judge rejected her argument, saying that being slapped and yelled at doesn't justify torture and murder. His judgment that she was not coerced derives from his conviction that her actions were unjustifiable; therefore she was morally responsible. In many situations, the judgment that someone was coerced or had no choice depends on whether we think the person was justified in acting as he or she did.

Offers and Threats

Both offers and threats are proposals that provide an external influence or impetus to action. Yet threats coerce, whereas offers generally do not. How can threats be distinguished from offers? The intuitive answer is that threats limit freedom, whereas offers enhance it; that one acts involuntarily in response to a threat, whereas one voluntarily accepts an offer; that the recipient of an offer is free to decline, whereas the recipient of a threat is not. Wertheimer characterizes the distinction between threats and offers this way: A threatens B by proposing to make B worse off relative to some baseline. A makes an offer when, if B does not accept A's proposal, B will be no worse off than in the relevant baseline position.

However, sometimes it seems that A's proposal can make B better off than he would have been, relative to his baseline situation, and still be coercive. Consider this example from Robert Nozick:

> *The Slave Case.* A beats B, his slave, each morning, for reasons having nothing to do with B's behavior. A proposes not to beat B the next morning, if B will do X, which is distasteful to him.

Assume that B would rather do X than get beaten. If we think of B's baseline as being set by what *normally happens* (call this the "statistical test"), A is making an offer (noncoercive). B expects to be beaten each morning, and relative to that expectation, A is proposing to make B better off. However, we can also think of the baseline as being set by what is *morally required* (call this the "moral test"). Under the moral test, A is making a threat (coercive). For A is morally required not to beat B, and indeed, not to own slaves at all; relative to that baseline, A is proposing to make B worse off. In addition to the statistical and moral tests, Wertheimer says there is also a "phenomeno-logical test": how it seems to B. A's proposal may *feel like* a threat to B. Consider the following example:

> Each week, A calls B and asks her for a date. They have grown fond of each other, but they have not had sexual intercourse. After three months, A tells B that unless she has sexual intercourse with him, he will stop dating her.

Wertheimer comments that under the statistical and phenomenological tests, B may or may not regard A's proposal as a threat. "That would depend upon the history of their relationship and B's expectations."[10] Applying the moral test is complicated, but Wertheimer thinks that it is clear that B has no right to expect A to continue dating her, and dating her on B's preferred terms. Relative to that moral baseline, A's proposal is an offer.

It is by no means clear that Wertheimer has applied the moral test correctly. One might equally argue that A is not entitled to expect sexual intercourse from B and that it is wrong to insist on sex as a condition of continuing the relationship. Relative to that moral baseline, A's proposal is a threat. The correct application of the moral test would depend on factual details not given, such as the age of the parties, their views on the morality of extramarital sexual intercourse, and so forth.

Wertheimer maintains that it is because there are these different tests, all of which can be used to characterize A's proposal as an offer or a threat, that intuitions about the coerciveness of proposals often conflict. What looks like an offer may really be a threat. It depends on what test is used—and, I would add, how the test is applied—to set the baseline. Moreover, Wertheimer doesn't think there's any way to decide which is *the* correct test to determine the baseline. This often makes it difficult to say with any certitude that a proposal is coercive (and so objectionable). Consider the following intriguing example:

> *The Lecherous Millionaire:* B's child will die without expensive surgery which her insurance doesn't cover and for which the state will not pay. A, a millionaire, offers to pay for the surgery if B will agree to become his mistress.

Wertheimer says that this is an offer under either the statistical or the moral test: B does not expect A to pay for her child's surgery, nor is A morally required to do so.

Some philosophers argue that offers, as well as threats, can be coercive. Joel Feinberg argues that the Lecherous Millionaire's proposal is a "coercive offer" because it manipulates B's options in such a way that B has no choice but to comply or suffer an unacceptable alternative. Wertheimer responds that A also "manipulates" B's options when he offers her a job at three times her present salary. This may well be "an offer she cannot refuse," yet surely such an offer is not coercive. Moreover, what if it was the child's mother who proposed to the millionaire, knowing of his lecherous propensities, that she become his mistress if he will pay for the surgery? Surely that wouldn't be a coercive offer, Wertheimer says, so why is it coercive when A makes the offer to B? A's proposal may be "unseemly," according to Wertheimer, but it is not coercive, because it expands rather than reduces B's options.

It appears that, for Wertheimer, the phenomenological test is not really a test of coerciveness at all. The fact that someone feels threatened is not conclusive evidence, if it is evidence at all, that the proposal is coercive. The true test, for Wertheimer, is whether the recipient's options have been expanded or reduced. This bears further examination. Can an offer which expands one's options nevertheless be coercive? Consider the proposal made in the fairy tale *Rumpelstiltskin*. According to the story, the miller's daughter will be put to death if she doesn't spin a roomful of straw into gold. Twice Rumpelstiltskin saves the miller's daughter by spinning the straw into gold in return for trinkets she gives him. The third time, however, the miller's daughter has nothing left to give him. Rumpelstiltskin then offers to spin the straw into gold in return for her firstborn child. The girl reluctantly accepts.

Has the miller's daughter been coerced? Feinberg would say yes. The decision to give up her child is not one she makes freely or willingly or voluntarily. She makes it because otherwise she will be killed. Admittedly, the miller's daughter prefers relinquishing her child[11] to being put to death, but the fact that she prefers one alternative to the other doesn't prevent the offer from being coercive. The robbery victim also prefers giving up his money to being killed. What makes both of these examples cases of coercion is that the choosers reasonably see themselves as having no choice.

Wertheimer would say that the miller's daughter was not coerced because if she declines Rumpelstiltskin's offer, she will be no worse off than she was before the offer was made. Admittedly, she will be put to death, but she would have been put to death anyway, regardless of whether Rumpelstiltskin made his proposal. In Wertheimer's analysis, then, Rumpelstiltskin's offer (distasteful as it may be) expands the maiden's options, and therefore is noncoercive.

Is there a way to reconcile the persuasive intuition that there can be coercive offers (and that the offers made by the Lecherous Millionaire and Rumpelstiltskin are such offers) with Wertheimer's analysis of coercion? One possibility is to reconsider the moral baseline. Under the moral test, whether Rumpelstiltskin is making an offer or a threat will depend on whether Rumpelstiltskin has an obligation to spin the straw into gold for the miller's daughter. It might seem that he has no such obligation. Individuals are not generally obligated to do work for others, especially without compensation. However, morality requires that we help others when they will die otherwise and when giving the help is not terribly onerous. We might not want such moral obligations to be made into law, but it is certainly plausible that there are such obligations. On this basis, it could be argued that Rumpelstiltskin ought to help the miller's daughter, even though she has nothing left to give him, because she needs his help so desperately and helping her isn't terribly burdensome to him. Relative to that moral baseline, he is proposing to make her worse off. His proposal is therefore a threat and by definition coercive.

However, this move will not help us with the Lecherous Millionaire. His offer can be seen as a threat only if we maintain that the millionaire has a moral obligation to pay for the child's expensive surgery. It does not seem plausible to maintain that a person—even a very wealthy person—is morally required to lay out large sums of money to meet the medical expenses of strangers. What's objectionable about the millionaire's behavior is not that he fails to help someone he could have helped; rather, it is that he exploits the woman's desperate situation in a particularly nasty way. That his offer is exploitative is unquestionable. The question is whether such exploitation should be regarded as coercive (because, under the circumstances, the child's mother has no choice) or whether it should be regarded as noncoercive (because the millionaire does not create, but merely takes advantage of, the woman's plight). In my opinion, this is an example of a difference that does not make a moral difference, since—as the examples show—an exploitative (but not coercive) offer can be as morally reprehensible as a coercive one.

Incentives

Incentives, like threats, are ways of trying to get people to do things. Unlike threats, incentives are typically welcome offers that seem morally unobjectionable. Yet sometimes inducements and incentives are alleged to be coercive. For example, A offers B, who is desperately poor, a large sum of money for his kidney. Why is this thought to be coercive? It isn't just that B is being offered a lot of money; generous offers are not coercive. Perhaps the objection is that B's impoverished situation may make him unable fully to weigh the costs and benefits of the proposal. He may be inclined to weigh too heavily the short-term benefits of having the money, versus the long-term risks of not having an extra kidney. Offering a poor person money for a body part exploits or takes advantage of his poverty, but it is not clear that it forces or coerces him.

Incentives to do things that people ordinarily would not consider doing appear to be in the same category as exploitative offers. Whether they are coercive is unclear. However, even if they are not coercive, they may be morally impermissible. Only a detailed substantive analysis can determine this. To determine the morality of offering incentives requires that we have to ask other questions such as whether persons in such conditions make intelligent judgments about their interests. Does society have an obligation to provide them with better alternatives? If society has not provided them with better alternatives, should such persons be allowed to improve their situations anyway?

The next section applies the above discussion of the concept of coercion to several issues: court-ordered birth control as a condition of probation, financial incentives for welfare mothers to use long-term contraception, the Dollar-a-Day program in Colorado, and the decision to offer Norplant in a Baltimore high school.

Applying the Concept of Coercion

People v. Johnson

Darlene Johnson was a twenty-seven-year-old African-American woman with a criminal record for check fraud, petty theft, disturbing the peace, battery, and burglary. At the time of her conviction for child abuse, she had four children and was pregnant with her fifth. Her eleven-year-old son was living with her mother and stepfather, and she had custody of her three daughters, aged three, five, and six.

On September 13, 1990, Johnson's stepfather contacted the police to report that she was physically abusing her children. The five- and six-year-old girls told the police that their mother and her boyfriend had beaten them with a belt—sometimes using the buckle end—and electrical cord. They had significant bruises on their backs, arms, necks, and legs. The state removed all of the children and placed them in foster care.

On December 13, Johnson pleaded guilty to three counts of inflicting corporal injury on children and appeared before Judge Howard Broadman, a judge known for his creative sentencing.[12] Because of her prior convictions Johnson could have been sentenced to six years in prison, but because her past crimes were unrelated to child abuse the judge felt imprisonment was inappropriate. Her application for probation was granted and her prison sentence was suspended for three years. Included in the conditions of probation were that she attend counselling and parenting programs; that she refrain from striking her children; and that she abstain from alcohol, tobacco, or drugs during her pregnancy. Finally, her probation was conditioned on her agreement to use Norplant for three years after she delivered. She was instructed to see her own doctor for insertion.

On January 10, 1991, Johnson's attorney moved for reconsideration of the Norplant condition, claiming that it violated her right to privacy and that by imposing such a condition the court was practicing medicine without a license. Johnson said that she had agreed out of fear of being sent back to prison and that she didn't know enough about Norplant to make an informed decision. Furthermore, she declared that she suffered from high blood pressure, heart murmurs, and diabetes, conditions that made her an unsuitable candidate for Norplant.

Judge Broadman denied the motion, maintaining that Johnson had given her informed consent to Norplant and that the terms of her probation were reasonably related to the compelling state interest in reformation, rehabilitation, and public safety. Acknowledging that the Norplant condition did impinge upon her right to procreate, the judge noted that the right is not absolute and may be balanced against the need to prevent child abuse. Johnson appealed, but on the eve of oral arguments her probation was revoked after she tested positive for cocaine on three occasions. She was sent to a state prison for five years.

Probation and Coercion

Was the imposition of Norplant as a condition of probation coercive? To decide this, we must ask whether Johnson's consent was given freely and autonomously. Two factors are pertinent to answering this question: first, whether Johnson was given information about Norplant necessary for her informed consent, and second, whether the threat of prison is an external influence or pressure that deprives decisions of their autonomous character.

Despite Judge Broadman's ruling, it is clear that Johnson did not give anything remotely resembling informed consent. Judge Broadman gave Johnson virtually no information about Norplant, beyond telling her that it was like the pill. She was not informed that the drug is not advised for women with diabetes or that some doctors will not prescribe Norplant for women with heart disease, blood clots, or high blood pressure. She was not told of any side effects of Norplant. In sum, she received none of the counselling recommended by Wyeth-Ayerst Laboratories (Norplant's American manufacturer), nor was she given the recommended thorough physical examination to screen for conditions that would contraindicate the use of Norplant. Nor was she given a chance to reflect on her decision or to consult with her lawyer. A decision made in such utter ignorance cannot be considered free or autonomous.

Suppose Judge Broadman had provided Ms. Johnson with more information about Norplant. What if he had made the order contingent upon her consent given after she had consulted with her doctor? Some would argue that she would still not have given genuine informed consent because her consent was based on the fear of going to jail. However, this is true of all probation conditions. Defendants agree to them because they want to avoid being sent to jail. Probation conditions thus meet Wertheimer's "choice prong": defendants have "no reasonable alternative" but to agree. If this makes probation conditions coercive, then probation itself is problematic, not just birth control as a condition of probation. Critics of Judge Broadman's sentence, however, have not objected to probation in general but only to the imposition of Norplant.

Opposition to Judge Broadman's sentence in particular, and not probation in general, can be explained if we remember that in Wertheimer's analysis coercion involves *two* tests, each of which is necessary. All probation conditions fulfill the choice prong, but what about the proposal prong? The proposal prong stipulates that the proposal is *wrongful* independent of its deprivation of free choice. To call a proposal wrongful is not merely to claim that there are objections to it. For example, there could be decisive utilitarian objections to a social policy. Such a policy would be a bad idea but not necessarily wrongful. To call a proposal wrongful implies that the proposer has no right to make it; that the very making of the proposal violates the rights of the person to whom it is made. Wrongful proposals includes ones that violate fundamental rights or due process, or discriminate against individuals on specious grounds.

It seems clear that the institution of probation does not qualify as a wrongful proposal and so probation conditions in general are not coercive. However, it could be argued that imposing Norplant *is* wrongful and that this differs from typical probation conditions such as restricting travel or freedom of association, even though these are both constitutionally protected rights. The difference is that Norplant is a medical treatment. It is specially wrong, it may be said, to impose invasive medical treatment as a condition of probation. The wrongfulness derives in part from a conception of the doctor-patient relationship, which is supposed to be based on good faith and mutual trust. In addition, the imposition of Norplant requires bodily invasion and has the potential for harmful side effects and contraindications. These features distinguish the imposition of forced medical treatment from other probation conditions. It is doubtful that someone could be sentenced to donate bone marrow or a pint of blood, even if such donation were plausibly related to a legitimate aim of probation such as rehabilitation. Note that these arguments are not based on the wrongfulness of restricting the probationer's fertility (an argument which is vulnerable to the counterargument that a prison term also restricts fertility), but rather on the special wrongfulness of administering punishment that violates the doctor-patient relationship, involves bodily invasion, and has potentially harmful side effects.

There are other serious problems with such sentences which merit consideration. For example, issues of race and class cannot be ignored. The women who are targeted for forced use of contraception—in particular, Norplant—are most often poor women and women of color. Ms. Johnson's prosecution and sentence were very likely influenced by her race.

> A recent Florida study found that black women are ten times more likely than white women to be referred for prosecution for substance abuse while pregnant, even though a comparable percentage of women of both races have been documented as using harmful drugs. Child abuse prosecutions are similarly influenced by race. It follows, therefore, that when women of color are convicted of child abuse or drug use while pregnant, and are subsequently forced to use Norplant, the decision is very likely to be racially motivated.[13]

In addition to race and class, gender is also an issue. Men procreate, men abuse children, yet it is only women whose procreative liberty is restricted. Darlene Johnson's boyfriend also allegedly beat her children, yet he was not even indicted, much less sentenced to use birth control. It might be argued that it is not so easy to mandate birth control for men, since there is no male equivalent of Norplant. However, judges have been willing to require that

women—but not men—consent to sterilization, even though vasectomy is
an available option. In January 1993, a Tennessee woman and her husband
were convicted of molesting the woman's two sons. They were each sentenced
to ten years in prison, but the judge said he would give them probation if
the *woman* would consent to a tubal ligation. The judge's offer did not require
her husband to be sterilized. The *New York Times* called the order "sexism at
its most flagrant":

> If he [Judge Brown] *really* believed that sterilization was sound punishment
> for molestation, shouldn't he have given the husband the same choice
> he gave the wife? Since when is it only women who are responsible
> for pregnancy?[14]

An issue relating to discrimination concerns contraception and religious
beliefs. Some religions (e.g., Roman Catholicism) prohibit the use of contraceptives. Women who are offered a choice between prison and contraception
are thus forced to choose between their freedom and their religion. Mandatory
use of Norplant may therefore violate the First Amendment.

In addition to informed consent and discrimination, mandated birth control
is likely to create problems with procedural due process. Due process is
violated when a court imposes a sentence that is vague or indefinite. The
probationer must be able to tell whether she is conforming with the probation
condition, and the court must be able to determine whether she has violated
its command. In addition, probation conditions must be one with which the
probationer is able to comply.[15]

Sometimes judges have ordered convicted child abusers "not to conceive."
Such orders are so vague as to violate due process. Is the order intended to
require the probationer to abstain from having sex? In *Johnson* and other cases,
the judges expressly noted that the sentences were not intended to interfere
with the defendants' rights to sexual expression. However, if courts do not
intend to mandate abstinence, an order not to conceive demands the impossible,
because no contraceptive method is 100% effective. Perhaps the order is
intended as requiring a good faith effort to avoid conception. However, this
is also indefinite and vague. There may be medical reasons why a woman
cannot use a very reliable form of contraception such as the pill or Norplant.
Her doctor may recommend against an IUD out of concern for future fertility.
If she faithfully uses a diaphragm and becomes pregnant anyway (the failure
rate is about ten percent), has she violated her probation? And how does a
court intend to monitor her use of such methods to determine compliance?

Mandating a specific form of birth control such as Norplant avoids the
problem of violating procedural due process. To comply with the probation

condition, the probationer need only have Norplant implanted and leave it in for the requisite period of time. Because Norplant is inserted in the upper arm, compliance can be determined without invading her privacy. If she should become pregnant, it would clearly be due to product failure, not to any lapse on her part.

However, Norplant is not for every woman. It has a range of side effects which make it unacceptable to some women. Moreover, women who smoke heavily, experience abnormal vaginal bleeding, blood clots, or any circulation or heart problems or liver disease, or who have had breast cancer or any condition for which they were treated with hormones are strongly advised against using Norplant. Women who have diabetes, high blood pressure, migraines or frequent headaches, depression, epilepsy, or gall bladder or kidney disease should consider Norplant use with extreme caution. To mandate Norplant for a woman who has one of these conditions, especially if her doctor advises against it, would violate every principle of informed consent and the right to refuse medical treatment.

Thus judges who wish to prevent convicted child abusers from having babies are caught between a rock and a hard place. As Arthur puts it:

> If a court complies with standards of due process by prescribing the contraceptive method to be used with clarity and precision, it may violate a probationer's right to give informed consent before receiving medical treatment. However, if a court chooses the less intrusive path and orders a defendant to consult with her physician and freely select the method of birth control that she prefers, it runs the risk that (1) she will choose none, or (2) that her choice will create insurmountable procedural due process problems.[16]

The likelihood that informed consent to medical treatment will not be obtained; the bodily invasiveness; the damage to the doctor-patient relationship; the potential for discrimination based on race, gender, or religion; and the violation of procedural due process—all of these make a powerful case for regarding the imposition of Norplant as a condition of probation wrongful. Thus such sentences fulfill both prongs and are properly denounced as coercive. Even if one takes the position that mandated birth control is no more coercive than other probation conditions, these additional objections are decisive reasons for rejecting mandated birth control as a condition of probation. I conclude that despite the legitimate concern with a rising tide of child abuse judges should not impose birth control as a condition of probation. At the same time, drug and psychological counselors as well as teachers of parenting classes will undoubtedly and properly urge women who are not yet capable of caring for themselves to get their lives in order before having more children. To do this, they will need access to substance abuse programs and contraception as well as protection from abusive husbands and boyfriends who force or intimidate them into sexual relations without contraceptives.

Financial Incentives for Using Birth Control

After Norplant was approved in December 1990, states moved rapidly to add Norplant to their Medicaid programs. All states except Massachusetts now reimburse poor women for all or part of the cost of Norplant. In 1991, a new kind of assistance program appeared: offering a cash bonus to women on public assistance if they use birth control (usually Norplant). In Kansas, a bill was introduced in 1991 that would have provided any woman on public assistance with a one-time grant of $500 for getting Norplant implanted, as well as $50 a year for each year she kept it in. Representative David Duke introduced a bill in 1991 that would have given Louisiana women on public assistance $100 a year if they used Norplant. It was amended in committee to provide $100 a year to any woman on public assistance who used any method of birth control, including abstinence. It was amended to remove cash incentives for the use of contraception. The final version of the bill simply provided that Norplant would be given free of charge to women on public assistance.

In Mississippi, a bill was introduced in 1992 that would have required women with four or more biological children to have Norplant implanted in order to be eligible to receive state assistance. In Tennessee, a bill was introduced in 1992 that would have provided a payment of $500 to women on public assistance if they agreed to be implanted with Norplant and additional payments of $50 annually at checkup time to ensure that the drug was still working. A similar bill was introduced in the state of Washington. All of these bills were either defeated or (more commonly) died in committee.

A bill is pending in Ohio that would provide a new welfare mother with a one-time payment of $1,000 and would increase her monthly cash assistance to 150% of her base subsidy if she is sterilized by tubal ligation. If she agreed to have a long-acting contraceptive such as Depo-Provera or Norplant, she would get a $500 payment and a 10% increase of her base subsidy every six months until it reached the 150% level. Under the bill's provisions, the welfare mother would be required to identify the father of the child. He could elect to pay child support, perform community service work, be sterilized and receive $1,000, or be sent to prison for two years. Also, a new welfare mother would have to pass a test prepared by the state Department of Human Services to show she has appropriate parenting skills. The newborn of a person who refuses to take the test or who fails could be placed with relatives or in a foster home. Under the bill, the child could be put up for adoption if the parent doesn't pass within a year.[17]

It is difficult to imagine anyone dreaming up such a cruel law. Even if we had reason to think that tests could be devised that would reliably indicate which individuals will be neglectful or abusive parents—which is very dubious—it would be outrageous to remove a newborn simply because its mother failed the test. She might have difficulty reading or comprehending the questions. She might not speak English well. She might simply have been nervous. Children are harmed when they are taken from their mothers and when they are put in foster care, especially an overburdened foster care system. Taking a newborn away from a mother who wants to keep it should be a last resort. Moreover, if society wants to ensure that children are cared for by people with adequate parenting skills, why focus on poor people? Child abuse exists in all classes and income levels. It is discriminatory to single out women on public assistance and force them to take tests to demonstrate their parenting skills or else lose their babies.

Leaving aside the Ohio bill, with its nightmarish conditions, are Norplant bonus programs in general coercive? Or are they a logical extension of other kinds of incentive programs such as those that offer incentives for welfare recipients to stay in school? In Ohio, for example, an experimental program paid teenage mothers on welfare a bonus of sixty-two dollars a month if they attended school. It deducted sixty-two dollars a month from their monthly checks if they skipped classes or dropped out. Researchers found that 61% of the teenage mothers already in school remained enrolled when they were offered incentives, as opposed to 51% who were not offered incentives. Among those who had already dropped out of school, 47% returned to classes under the incentive program, compared with 33% who were not given an incentive. Senator Daniel Patrick Moynihan was so impressed with the results that he is urging the Clinton Administration to offer the same education incentives nationwide.[18]

Most commentators have no objection to educational incentives. It is pointed out that financial gain motivates the poor like everyone else and that there is nothing wrong with such incentives. If it is acceptable to offer tax breaks to the rich to get them to act in socially responsible ways (e.g., donating their art to museums rather than selling it), it is equally acceptable to offer cash incentives to young mothers to get them to stay in school.

By contrast, many regard incentives to persuade women on public assistance not to get pregnant as coercive. They argue that women are not free to reject the extra money and that it is intrinsically wrongful to ask them to curb their fertility. Let us look more closely at the arguments against this kind of incentive.

The Unconstitutional Conditions Doctrine

"The doctrine of unconstitutional conditions holds that government may not grant a benefit on the condition that the beneficiary surrender a constitutional right, even if the government may withhold that benefit altogether."[19] The doctrine emerged during the *Lochner* era[20] to protect the economic liberties of foreign corporations and private truckers. It reemerged under the Warren Court to protect personal liberties of speech, religion, and privacy. For example, the doctrine was applied to hold that the government may not condition tax exemptions or government jobs on political silence and may not condition unemployment benefits on acceptance of work on one's sabbath day.

A law that forced women to use birth control would clearly be unconstitutional. The right of privacy gives individuals the right to use or not use contraceptives without government intervention. If the government cannot compel women to use birth control, then it would seem that the unconstitutional conditions doctrine does not allow the government to condition a benefit such as a cash bonus on the use of birth control.

However, substantial uncertainty remains about the rationale for and application of the doctrine. The Supreme Court has repeatedly suggested that the problem with unconstitutional conditions is their coercive effect. However, we earlier distinguished offers, which are supposedly not coercive, from threats, which are. The question, then, is whether monetary incentives to use birth control are offers or threats. The answer to that question depends on whether the proposal makes the intended recipient worse off. It might be argued that Norplant bonus programs do not make anyone worse off, since while those who choose to participate are given extra benefits, the benefits of those who opt not to take the offer are not reduced. They remain in the same economic position they had prior to the offer. In Wertheimer's analysis, such an offer appears not to be coercive.

David Coale argues that offering such a bonus does make those who do not take it worse off and thus burdens the constitutional right not to take Norplant. He writes:

> . . . poor women who do not take Norplant must forego $1000 in consumption possibilities. Women who do not take Norplant then suffer the harm of a reduction in economic status compared to women who do take the drug. That reduction affects their self-esteem, which then changes almost every aspect of their lives.[21]

Unless women agree to waive their constitutional right to reproduce, they are threatened with economic loss compared to what others receive. Put this way, Norplant bonuses look coercive. But is this a plausible interpretation?

It seems to prove too much. The government attempts to influence behavior of various kinds through tax breaks and incentives: to get people to donate to charity, to save money, to join retirement plans. Such plans make some people comparatively better off than those who opt not to participate, but it is not plausible that the non-participants are thereby harmed or made worse off by the program.

Coale might respond that it isn't the difference in income itself that is objectionable, but rather the impact on self-esteem. It is unlikely that someone who decides to keep an art object and forego a tax advantage will suffer a loss in self-esteem—quite the opposite. By contrast, having to buy one's children food, clothing, or toys that are substandard and decidedly inferior to those of other children might be a severe blow to one's self-esteem as a parent and provider. A woman who declines Norplant is thus exposed to a threat to her self-esteem, which she can avoid only by waiving her right to reproduce. At the same time, the blow to self-esteem caused by a lower comparative income might be offset by the increase in self-esteem from having another child. It remains unclear whether programs that offer women bonuses to get Norplant make those who refuse it worse off and are therefore coercive.

Sullivan argues that coercion cannot serve as the ordering principle of unconstitutional conditions doctrine. Because coercion is an inescapably normative concept, we would have to agree on the appropriate baselines in order to be able to distinguish offers from threats. "Any such effort, however, is especially problematic in the context of unconstitutional conditions, which arise against the backdrop of a constitutional jurisprudence in which most redistribution is permissible and few affirmative obligations on government are imposed."[22] Since the government does not have to offer any welfare benefits at all, it is impossible to construct or identify a normative baseline that would distinguish threats from offers.

In any event, Sullivan thinks that focusing on coercion alone misses the point:

> There is good reason to turn elsewhere in a search for the rationale of unconstitutional conditions doctrine, both because the necessary baselines are elusive, once government benefits in this context are conceded to be gratuitous, and because government, which differs significantly from any given individual, can burden rights to autonomy through means other than coercion. Coercion thus begins rather than ends the inquiry.[23]

According to Sullivan, unconstitutional conditions cases raise issues of equality as well as liberty. These cases inherently classify potential beneficiaries into two groups: those who comply with the condition, and thereby get better treatment, and those who do not. ". . . [B]ackground inequalities of wealth and resources necessarily determine one's bargaining position in relation to government . . . the poor may have nothing to trade but their liberties."[24] Coale makes a similar point when he says, "A society that professes a commitment to universal liberty suffers when its weakest members are surcharged to enjoy those liberties."[25]

The Supreme Court acknowledged this problem in its decision in *Skinner v. Oklahoma*[26] when it invalidated, on equal protection grounds, a state requirement of sterilization for recidivist thieves but not embezzlers. Sullivan suggests that this decision holds that some rights (such as the right to procreate) are too important to be reserved for selected privileged groups. Where rights have this character, conditions on benefits that affect their exercise pose a similar danger of hierarchy:

> For example, conditioning welfare benefits on contribution of body organs to a public organ bank, or aid to mothers with dependent children on their service as surrogate mothers in a public program to remedy infertility, would unconstitutionally create a donor caste. This argument does not depend on either the view that such exchanges are "coerced" by the desperation of poverty, or the view that body parts or gestational services are generally inalienable.[27]

Of course, Norplant bonuses are not conditioned on anything so drastic as organ donation or serving as a surrogate mother. They merely require women to suspend procreation temporarily. Nor do such programs condition welfare benefits on compliance; they offer bonuses instead. Nevertheless, the fact that such programs target the poor raises concerns about creating an impermissible hierarchy. Sullivan suggests a "strict scrutiny" test for "any government benefit condition whose primary purpose or effect is to pressure recipients to alter a choice about exercise of a preferred constitutional liberty in a direction favored by government."[28] This does not mean that government could never burden a preferred liberty, since some burdens may ultimately survive strict scrutiny. The question would be whether the state's interests to be achieved by imposing the condition are sufficiently compelling to justify the burden on the preferred liberty.

What are the state's interests in offering Norplant bonuses? Obviously, saving the state money by reducing the number of children on welfare is a prime motivation, but this interest is not sufficiently compelling to justify restricting a fundamental right. Another reason is offered by Coale:

> The most visible reason is growing discontent with the current welfare system. Decades of "antipoverty" programs have been widely criticized for failing to elevate living standards and instead creating an intergenera-

tional cycle of welfare dependency. Those critics advocate reforms that would encourage welfare recipients to break that cycle. Examples of reforms include incentives for welfare recipients to attend school and restructuring AFDC benefits to discourage large families. Proposals to encourage Norplant use seem a natural outgrowth of this movement.[29]

The attempt to help people out of poverty is certainly a legitimate, perhaps even a compelling, state interest. It is not clear, however, that the state can try to achieve this goal through incentives for using birth control. It can be argued that linking Norplant to welfare benefits goes beyond legitimate attempts toward helping the poor improve their lives. Providing people with information about birth control, making contraceptives accessible and affordable (or even free), paying for abortion as well as childbirth—all of these activities are acceptable because they enhance individual choice. Offering fairly large sums of money to use Norplant is a different matter. A bonus of $500 to a woman on public assistance may mean the difference between the rent getting paid or not; $50 may mean the children have shoes or Christmas presents. Norplant bonuses specifically target poor women by offering them relatively large sums of money in order to influence and pressure their procreative decisions. Even if such programs are not clearly coercive, they pose a threat to the values of autonomy and equality and should be rejected for these reasons.

Does this mean that financial incentives for procreative decisions are always improper? Not necessarily. Consider the Dollar-a-Day program sponsored by Planned Parenthood in Denver, whose goal is to reduce the repeat pregnancy rate for teens, mostly black and Hispanic, who have become pregnant before the age of sixteen. The program requires girls to come to one meeting a week, where they receive their seven dollars, paid out for symbolic reasons in one dollar bills. Girls who become pregnant must drop out of the group.

After five years, the program was judged a success. Only 17% of the girls in the program became pregnant; this compares very favorably to a 50% risk of repeat pregnancy within two years for girls who have become pregnant before age sixteen. In addition, the program is claimed to have saved Colorado in excess of a quarter of a million dollars in welfare and Medicaid payments. Despite these advantages, President Faye Wattleton and a majority of the board of Planned Parenthood Federation of America denounced the program as "coercive." Paying teenagers not to get pregnant, they felt, went against the organization's long-standing and deeply held policies advocating reproductive choice and individual rights.

Is the Dollar-a-Day program coercive? It seems clear that the choice prong is not satisfied. The girls are not threatened or forced or pressured into avoiding pregnancy. Rather, a small financial incentive is offered—enough to get the girls into the program, but not so much that they have no reasonable alternative but to join. If they decide not to join, they are not thereby made worse off.

I noted above that, unlike Wertheimer, Feinberg thinks that there can be "coercive offers," like that made by the Lecherous Millionaire. Feinberg regards the Millionaire's offer to pay for the child's operation in exchange for sexual favors from the mother as coercive—even though the offer expanded the mother's options—because she had no choice but to comply or else suffer an unacceptable alternative (the child's death). By contrast, Wertheimer thinks that the offer is morally offensive and exploitative but not coercive. With either theory, the Dollar-a-Day program is not coercive. Nor can the program be considered exploitative because whatever financial benefits it has for the state, its primary benefit is to the girls themselves, who are likely to remain in poverty if they have a child, or especially two children, before the age of twenty. Getting teenage girls to delay pregnancy is not like getting them to give up kidneys or become surrogate mothers—something they might choose under the pressure of poverty and regret later on.

The second prong is satisfied if offering financial incentives to get people to avoid pregnancy is wrongful—that is, something the state has no right to do. It is likely that Planned Parenthood's opposition to financial incentives for birth control and its labeling of the program as coercive is based on its perception that such incentives are inherently wrong. The fundamental philosophy of Planned Parenthood is that reproductive choices should be made by individuals in accordance with their own values and goals and that any attempt to pressure or influence such choices, particularly with monetary inducements, is wrong. This is reflected in Planned Parenthood's mission statement:

> Planned Parenthood believes in the fundamental right of each individual, throughout the world, to manage his or her fertility, regardless of the individual's income, marital status, age, national origin, or residence. We believe that reproductive self-determination must be voluntary and preserve the individual's right to privacy. We further believe that such self-determination will contribute to an enhancement of the quality of life, strong family relationships, and population stability.

However, it is doubtful that small financial incentives infringe on self-determination or compromise the individual's voluntary choice. Moreover, to oppose monetary incentives on the ground that they illegitimately influence teens to avoid pregnancy is to ignore the psychological and peer pressures to *get* pregnant placed on the girls targeted by the program. Some, desperate for love, become pregnant because their boyfriends, anxious to prove their masculinity by fathering as many children as possible, want them to. Others harbor entirely unrealistic hopes about what a baby will mean to their lives. They think that the baby will love them, not realizing that the baby needs all of their love and attention.

> Many of the girls in the target population had been physically or sexually abused by their mothers' boyfriends; even those who were not the victims of abuse exuded a sense of hopelessness and a profound lack of self-confidence. For some, having a child gave them something to look forward to.[30]

Although money is used to lure the girls to the meetings, it is ultimately the support they get from the other girls which enables them to resist the pressures to get pregnant. For some, shy about admitting they care about the group, the money is a face-saving mechanism. One board member emphasizes that Dollar-a-Day provides support otherwise lacking in the lives of these young women:

> If you can just get them [to avoid pregnancy] until they are 18 or 19 you've gone a long way. They are getting care and attention they've never had before. It's a different kind of attention than the kind they would get from a boyfriend.[31]

While the use of financial incentives raises the potential for coercion or improper influence, the facts suggest that the Dollar-a-Day program is reasonably seen as liberty-enhancing rather than as liberty-limiting. While programs of (much larger) incentives for women on public assistance to use birth control can be criticized as threatening autonomy and equality, the Dollar-a-Day program promotes these values. Characterizing the program as coercive is inaccurate and misleading.

Offering Long-Term Birth Control in the Schools

Baltimore, which has one of the highest rates of teenage pregnancy in the country, was the first city in the nation to provide Norplant in a school-based clinic. In 1990, Norplant was introduced into the Laurence G. Paquin School, a high school for pregnant teenagers and teenaged mothers, all of whom are at high-risk for another pregnancy. Its critics contend that encouraging long-term birth control—especially among low-income black women—is paternalistic and racist. Melvin Tuggle, a black Baltimore minister, calls the plan "genocide."[32]

Nan Marie Astone, assistant professor of population dynamics at The Johns Hopkins School of Hygiene and Public Health, characterizes the Norplant program at the Paquin School as a "prototypical public health intervention."[33] While opposition to such programs typically comes from conservative traditionalists who oppose them on moral grounds, some liberal activists have also objected to the program.

> Specifically, they question whether earlier Norplant safety studies are applicable to inner-city teenagers, many of whom smoke, are in poor health, and have limited access to health care. African-American community leaders have similar concerns—which should come as no surprise since African-Americans, like women, have a history of being used as guinea pigs by the medical establishment.[34]

The National Black Women's Health Project has expressed serious reservations about Norplant. President Julia R. Scott says that while the group supports the development of new technologies that are safe and improve the reproductive choices of women, and acknowledges the serious negative consequences of teenage pregnancy, it remains apprehensive whenever government targets a particular group of women (here, teenagers, but poor women generally) for one kind of contraceptive. The group

> . . . recognizes the potential for coercion and racially discriminatory use of long-acting contraceptives given the rich history in this country regarding the violations of the principles of informed consent (i.e., the *Relf v. Weinberger* (1973) case involving two black teen girls who were sterilized at a federally funded clinic in Alabama without the knowledge of the girls or their parents).[35]

These concerns, legitimate as they are, do not apply to the Paquin School Norplant Program. The principles of informed consent are scrupulously observed. The young women are counselled about the different contraceptive options. If they decide they want Norplant, they are counselled about the possible side effects. A complete physical examination with lab work is done prior to Norplant insertion. Although the Maryland Minor Consent Law allows teens to get Norplant without parental consent, the program's goal is to have as much positive parental involvement as possible. Usually a parent or guardian is present at the counselling session and often at the insertion too. However, according to a sheet giving details of the program, parental coercion—that is, a parent insisting that his/her daughter be implanted—is not tolerated. "It must be the adolescent's decision to have Norplant inserted." Moreover, Norplant is never "pushed" on teens. It is offered as one contraceptive option among many, and only after extensive counseling. According to Peter Beilenson, Baltimore city commissioner of public health, who initiated the program, "There is absolutely no promotion of one kind of contraceptive over another." Beilenson characterizes the opposition to the Norplant program at Paquin as "a small vocal minority of the religious right—Farrakhan Muslims" and says that the program has "overwhelming support" from the teens and their parents.[36] He questions why the views of a minority of male ministers should take precedence over the wishes of young women and their parents.

If the Paquin School program is neither coercive nor racially discriminatory nor violates informed consent, is it problem-free? Not necessarily. Another concern about Norplant is that it fails to protect against HIV infection and other sexually transmitted diseases (STDs). According to Beilenson, this is a real problem, and one which they try to combat at the Paquin School with extensive counseling. A small study was conducted which showed that, on the basis of self-reporting, backed up by testing for sexually transmitted diseases, the teens who opted for Norplant are using condoms at least as much as they had before they got Norplant. The introduction of Norplant has not decreased the rate of condom use and may have increased it because of counselling which emphasizes that protection from pregnancy is not protection from disease. Beilenson speculates that, freed from worry about contraception, the girls may be concentrating more on protecting themselves from disease. In any event, there is no reason to object specifically to Norplant as failing to protect against disease, since this is a feature of all contraceptive methods except condoms used with contraceptive foam.

Conclusion

Long-acting contraceptives like Norplant which are easy to monitor and do not require user-compliance clearly have a potential for coercive use. However, the charge of coercion is sometimes unwarranted, as in the politically motivated criticisms of Norplant in the Paquin School clinic. The potential for coercion is greater where there are financial incentives, as in the Dollar-a-Day program, because there is the risk that financial pressures will force individuals to make reproductive choices contrary to their own values and preferences. However, it seems extremely unlikely that small amounts of money could constitute such pressure. In addition, the psychosocial pressures *toward* teenage pregnancy are very strong among some groups, despite the fact that teenage childbearing has a very negative impact on the lives of the young women and their children. Small financial incentives, combined with other sorts of encouragement, can counteract these harmful influences.

It is more difficult to determine whether incentives paid to women on public assistance who get Norplant are coercive. Those who think they are not coercive point to the fact that the women who opt not to have Norplant are no worse off for refusing it than they would be if there were no incentive program. The program thus expands rather than contracts their options. Those who think they are coercive maintain that poor women have no choice but to accept Norplant or else suffer an unacceptable alternative—that is, going without desperately needed money. This dispute may be unresolvable if, as Wertheimer and Sullivan maintain, there isn't any way to decide which is the correct baseline, and therefore no way to decide whether the proposal is coercive. However, coercion is not the only possible objection. Focussing entirely on whether such programs are coercive may mask other important objections to such programs—the targeting of vulnerable groups and the creation and reinforcement of inequality.

The clearest example of the coercive use of Norplant is mandatory birth control as a condition of probation. Such sentences are not coercive solely because defendants agree to them in order to avoid going to jail; all probation conditions share this feature. However, because such sentences are potentially discriminatory and violate religious freedom, due process, and norms of informed consent, they are morally and legally objectionable. Calling them coercive alludes to the features that make such probation conditions wrongful.

NOTES

1. Some may be affronted by the implicit assumption that contraception is solely a woman's problem. Ideally, of course, contraception would be the responsibility of both partners. Unfortunately, in the world as it is today, it is primarily women who are adversely affected by unwanted pregnancies.

2. Women's Legal Defense Fund, *Legislation and Litigation Involving Norplant* (Washington, D.C.: Women's Legal Defense Fund, June 1992).

3. At least ten states have considered legislation regarding Norplant in 1993, but so far the only bill that has passed is one introduced by Representative Flowers in Illinois, which provides that a court may *not* impose a sentence that requires the defendant to use any form of birth control.

4. Tamar Lewin, "Five-Year Contraceptive Implant Seems Headed for Wide Use," *New York Times*, 29 November 1991, A1.

5. Barbara Feringa, Sarah Iden, and Allan Rosenfield, "Norplant: Potential for Coercion," in *Dimensions of New Contraceptives: Norplant and Poor Women*, ed. Sarah E. Samuels and Mark D. Smith (Henry J. Kaiser Family Foundation, 1992), 58.

6. Are legal sanctions, taxation, and mandated immunization coercive? On the one hand, they clearly do restrict freedom and force people to act in ways they would prefer not to act or else suffer unacceptable consequences. If this feature suffices to render institutions and policies coercive, then not all coercion is morally objectionable. On the other hand, the analysis of coercion on which I will rely in this paper maintains that only *wrongful* proposals are coercive. Since legal sanctions, taxation, and mandated immunization are presumably justifiable—i.e., not wrongful—they are not coercive. With either interpretation, the important point is that it is not necessarily wrong to force people to act in certain ways or be subject to unacceptable consequences.

7. Alan Wertheimer, *Coercion* (Princeton, N.J.: Princeton University Press, 1987).

8. See, for example, David Zimmerman, "Coercive Wage Offers," *Philosophy & Public Affairs* 10 (1981): 121–45.

9. See Kathleen M. Sullivan, "Unconstitutional Conditions," *Harvard Law Review* 102: 7 (1989): 1413–506.

10. Wertheimer, *Coercion*, 211.

11. More precisely, she prefers *promising* to relinquish her firstborn child to being put to death. That promise will not have to be fulfilled until some time in the future, and anything could happen. She might not have a child, Rumpelstiltskin might die, or he might forget her promise. Admittedly, it is possible that the king might not carry out his threat to put her to death if the straw isn't spun into gold, but the king's threat is much more immediate and, for that reason, more certain.

12. Stacey L. Arthur, "The Norplant Prescription: Birth Control, Woman Control, or Crime Control?" *University of California Los Angeles Law Review* 40 (1992): 34.

13. Julia R. Scott, "Norplant and Women of Color," in *Norplant and Poor Women*, 46.

14. *New York Times*, 10 February 1993.

15. Arthur, "Norplant Prescription," 84.

16. Arthur, "Norplant Prescription," 99.

17. Ohio House Bill 343, 1993.

18. Jason DeParle, "Ohio Welfare Bonuses Keep Teen-age Mothers in School," *New York Times*, 12 April 1993, A14.

19. Sullivan, "Unconstitutional Conditions," 1415.

20. *Lochner v. New York*, 198 U.S. 45 (1905). In the "Lochner era," the Supreme Court struck down much economic welfare legislation as a violation of the due process clause of the Fourteenth Amendment.

21. David S. Coale, "Norplant Bonuses and the Unconstitutional Conditions Doctrine," *Texas Law Review* 71 (1992): 208.

22. Sullivan, "Unconstitutional Conditions," 1450.

23. Ibid., 1456.

24. Ibid., 1497–98.

25. Coale, "Norplant Bonuses," 210.

26. 316 U.S. 535 (1942).

27. Sullivan, "Unconstitutional Conditions," 1498–99.

28. Ibid., 1499–500.

29. Coale, "Norplant Bonuses," 196–97.

30. Nancy Kates, "Buying Time: The Dollar-a-Day Program" (case study written at the request of Professor Marc Roberts for use at the Kennedy School of Government, Harvard University, 1990), 2.

31. Ibid., 11.

32. Barbara Kantrowitz and Pat Wingert, "The Norplant Debate," *Newsweek*, 15 February 1993, 37.

33. Nan Marie Astone, "Thinking About Teenage Childbearing," *Report from the Institute for Philosophy and Public Policy* 13: 3 (1993): 8–13.

34. Ibid., 12.

35. Julia R. Scott, "A Dangerous Combination: Norplant and Teens," *Health and Fitness: Walking for Wellness* 1 (1993).

36. Peter Beilenson, telephone conversation with author, 27 May 1993.

JOHN A. ROBERTSON

Norplant and Irresponsible Reproduction

Norplant offers safe and effective contraception for up to five years, thus increasing options for women seeking to control their fertility. Yet shortly after FDA approval in 1990, proposals surfaced to have Norplant implanted in child abusers, welfare mothers, and teenagers. Because the contraceptive effect of Norplant is reversible at any time, it appeared to offer an acceptable technological solution for harmful or irresponsible reproduction.

However, the notion of state intervention to limit reproduction is anathema to many people. If procreation is a basic right, then people must be allowed to reproduce as they wish and the consequences tolerated, just as the consequences of free speech or the due process rights of criminals must be tolerated. Still, the possibility of temporary interference with irresponsible reproduction is an attractive option. At the very least, this technology forces us to address issues of reproductive responsibility that have long been ignored. This chapter discusses irresponsible reproduction and the social policies which may be adopted to discourage it.[1]

The Norplant System

On December 10, 1990, the Food and Drug Administration approved Norplant for use in the United States.[2] The Norplant system of contraception consists of six flexible silastic matchstick-sized capsules that contain levonorgestrel, a synthetic progestin widely used in oral contraceptives. The capsules are inserted under the skin of the upper arm in a ten- to fifteen-minute procedure done with local anesthesia. Women can feel the implant under the skin, but it is not ordinarily visible.

Once implanted, the levonorgestrel slowly diffuses through the walls of the capsules into the bloodstream.[3] Norplant achieves contraception by suppressing ovulation, like contraceptive pills, and by thickening a woman's cervical mucus to impede passage of sperm into the uterus. The chance of becoming pregnant with Norplant averages less than 5% per year over five years, making the Norplant system the most effective contraceptive available except for permanent sterilization. Since it is estrogen-free, it can be used safely in women who are hypertensive or diabetic, who have migraine headaches, or who are over forty years old and smoke.

Norplant is also very convenient for users. Once implanted, nothing further need be done—a distinct advantage over barrier methods and the pill. The most common side effect is a disruption of menstrual patterns, with some women experiencing amenorrhea and others irregular bleeding. Some users also experience headaches, weight change, and acne. Current studies show, however, that when the chance of these effects is explained, 94% of women are satisfied with the implants, with 71% stating that they would use this method again.[4]

A major advantage is that Norplant's contraceptive effect is reversible at any time.[5] When the woman wishes to regain fertility, the capsules are removed under local anesthetic through a small incision in the skin. Within a week of removal, the level of levonorgestrel is almost undetectable in the bloodstream, and normal ovulation is soon restored.

The current cost of Norplant is $365, with an additional charge of $150-$650 for the insertion, counselling, and checkups. A $150-$300 fee for removal may also be charged. While the $365 price compares favorably with the cost of five years of oral contraceptives, that comparison does not take into account surgical fees for implantation and removal. Also, if removal occurs before five years, the cost advantage is lost. For women who tolerate the relatively minor side effects and who can afford it, it will be preferable to the inconvenience of taking an oral contraceptive or using barrier methods. However, it provides no protection against sexually transmitted disease.

Access to Norplant

A major problem with Norplant is making the system available to women who cannot pay the relatively high, up-front cost. Wyeth-Ayerst, the distributor of the system, is charging both public and private providers $365 for the silastic tubes. While Medicaid will cover this fee for the medically indigent, low Medicaid reimbursement rates for insertion may deter some doctors from providing it. Also, there are millions of women who are not poor enough to qualify for Medicaid or rich enough to pay the full up-front cost of the device, which health insurance usually does not cover.[6] Private agencies such as Planned Parenthood will fill some of that gap, but many women who want the device may not be able to afford it. If women are to be guaranteed control over their fertility through contraception, long-acting contraceptives such as Norplant should be made available to all women who desire it.[7]

A related question concerns access by teenagers who are at risk of pregnancy. The issues are no different than those that arise with other contraceptives for teenagers. If parents approve and are willing to pay the cost, access is not a problem. In other cases, lack of information, the need for parental consent, and money will be a substantial barrier to teenage access. In addition, public programs to provide teenagers with Norplant will have to overcome perceptions that provision of contraceptives encourages sexual activity or is otherwise coercive.

Norplant Controversies

As a voluntary method of contraception that has met regulatory standards of safety and efficacy, Norplant presents no major ethical or legal issues beyond making it available to all women who want it and ensuring that women are informed of its side effects. Voluntary use by adolescents raises issues of parental consent and impact on nonmarital sexual activity, but these issues arise with any contraceptive use by minors.

Norplant has become controversial, however, because of attempts by judges, legislators, and others to require that certain women use Norplant to avoid reproduction that is considered socially irresponsible or harmful to children and society. Within a month of FDA approval, for example, a trial judge in California offered to release from prison a woman convicted of child abuse if she would consent to use of Norplant. Other judges have offered similar deals to women, and legislation authorizing involuntary insertion of Norplant in alchoholics and drug addicts who have given birth to children has been introduced in Washington state.[8]

Legislators have also been quick to offer Norplant to women on welfare. In 1991, a Kansas legislator introduced a bill that would pay $500 to any mother on welfare who had Norplant implanted and $50 a year to maintain it. David Duke introduced a similar bill in Louisiana with a $100 reward. A 1990 editorial in the the *Philadelphia Inquirer* proposed making use of Norplant a condition of welfare as a way to reduce the size of the "underclass."[9] In January 1993, the Governor of Maryland proposed that use of Norplant be made mandatory in certain cases.[10]

Mental health professionals have considered use of Norplant with retarded and mentally ill women who are at risk of sexual exploitation in residential facilities. Others have proposed that Norplant be required or offered to women who are HIV-infected and to women who are at risk for offspring with severe genetic disease. Still others would provide Norplant to teenagers at school clinics.[11] Proposals to have Norplant inserted in all girls at puberty have also surfaced.[12]

Reactions to such proposals have varied from enthusiastic approval to horror and outrage. Approval comes from those persons who believe that certain kinds of reproduction is irresponsible and that the state may take steps to discourage or even eliminate such irresponsibility, particularly with an easily reversible device such as Norplant. Others see proposals to offer, entice, or compel women to use Norplant as a violation of basic human rights—a racist or elitest response to problems that should be resolved by other means. Such an approach is especially dubious because women vary in their tolerance of Norplant's irregular bleeding and other side effects.

Whatever one's views about these proposals, it is clear that Norplant has succeeded in reintroducing a discourse of reproductive responsibility into public life. Because Norplant is easily inserted and fully reversible, it appears to be much less intrusive of personal rights and dignity than is compulsory sterilization. Moreover, many of the proposals are not directly coercive, but provide incentives for target groups to use Norplant. The result is a long overdue discussion of reproductive responsibility and the state's role in promoting such responsibility.

Reproductive Responsibility

I have elsewhere presented the case for recognition of both a moral and legal right to reproduce. Arguing that reproduction is important to individuals because of the personal and social meanings that surround it, I have concluded that decisions to reproduce should be viewed as presumptive rights that are subject to limitation only upon the showing of substantial harm to the interests of others. The development of Norplant now requires us to address what kinds of harm would constitute a sufficient basis for limitation of that right.

Any discussion of reproductive responsibility and government action to limit reproduction is a touchy subject, however.[13] The history of attempts to limit irresponsible reproduction is replete with abuse and discrimination. From 1920 to 1960 more than 60,000 "mental defectives" were forcibly sterilized on eugenic grounds, even though the risk of transmission of genetic disease was low and diagnostic errors of mental deficiency abounded.[14] Poor and minority women have also been sterilized without consent under both public and private programs well into the 1970s.[15] As a result, there is an extreme reluctance to even discuss the idea of irresponsible reproduction, much less propose coercive policies, for fear that it will be viewed as racism or lead to coercive state policies that will replicate earlier abuses.

Nevertheless, it is essential that conversations about reproductive responsibility take place. Reproduction always has potential moral significance because it leads to the birth of another person whose needs for love, nurturing, and resources have to be met. Clearly, one can act responsibly or irresponsibly in reproducing because of the impact that one's actions will have on offspring and others. A dialogue about the circumstances that make reproduction desirable or undesirable, advised or ill-advised, responsible or irresponsible is needed to help us determine the parameters of morally and socially acceptable conduct and to guide or limit governmental action that affects reproductive choice.

Any judgment about the reproductive responsibility of individuals must pay attention to four issues: the importance of the reproduction in question to the person(s) reproducing; the ease or difficulty with which they could avoid that reproduction; the burdens that reproduction will cause resulting offspring; and the burdens or costs imposed on society and others.[16] Clarifying these parameters is necessary before they are applied to individual cases and questions of public policy are addressed.

Reproductive Interest

Reproduction is often said to be irresponsible because of the costs it imposes on others. Implicit in such a judgment is the assumption that the person reproducing has little or no reproductive interest to justify those costs. What counts as a reproductive interest? What distinctions can be made on this score?

An important issue here will be whether the persons will be involved in rearing resulting offspring. Although reproduction may occur without rearing, one reason why reproduction is highly valued is because of the rearing and family experiences which it makes possible. A person who reproduces but has no contact with offspring may have a lesser interest in reproduction than a person who reproduces with the intent to rear children. Whether the reproduction of either is undesirable will depend upon the costs imposed on offspring and society. However, in balancing those costs against the value of the reproductive experience, the capacity and likelihood of rearing is a relevant factor.

Given this parameter a man who fathers many children with different women but who has no contact with any of them and provides no support is more easily open to a charge of irresponsibility. At the opposite extreme would be cases where the person(s) reproducing is seeking to nurture and rear her offspring. Women infected with HIV, welfare mothers, and unmarried teenagers may fit this category. Although their reproduction may be undesirable because of consequences for offspring and the welfare system, they have substantial reproductive interests at stake when they also will rear their offspring. Because reproduction with rearing is presumptively protected, a correspondingly high level of harm will have to be shown to justify overriding their procreative freedom.

Other cases will fall in between these two extremes with many variations among them. Some persons may have minimal contact with offspring, rear intermittently, or require the assistance of other rearers. Some may rear fully but die while offspring are still young. Also relevant in assessing the value of the reproductive interest at stake will be whether the person has previously reproduced or will be able to reproduce in the future if the opportunity at issue is not used.

The key question in each case will be the value to the person and others of the precise reproductive experience that is occurring. Answering this question, however, will pose many problems beyond merely determining whether genetic reproduction *tout court* should be valued as much as genetic reproduction-cum-rearing. If the question is pushed, questions of the worth of the experience to the person will have to be faced and distinctions drawn based on previous and likely future reproductive experiences, expected life span, the amount of rearing, and the like. Because of these complications, it may not be possible as a practical matter in most cases to go beyond whether the person reproducing will be aware that they have reproduced and whether they will have contact with offspring.

Burdens of Avoiding Reproduction

Judgments of irresponsible reproduction will also have to factor in the ease or burdens of alternatives open to the person to avoid reproduction. Even if reproduction imposes high costs on others and the person has only a minimal reproductive interest at stake, a charge of irresponsiblity will fit only if the person has reasonable alternatives to reproduction. A person who could have been abstinent, used birth control, or terminated pregnancy would be acting irresponsibly if their failure to do so imposes high costs on others, particularly if they have no intention or ability to rear resulting offspring. On the other hand, if they have been raped, cannot remain abstinent, or birth control or abortion is dangerous, not available, or morally repugnant, then their responsibility is less.

The hard cases here will arise over whether alternatives to reproduction are reasonably available. For example, should a conscientious belief about the immorality of birth control or abortion justify actions that produce little or no significant reproductive experience and impose high costs on others? Must a woman insist that she or her partner use contraception? The lack of moral accountability for undesirable reproduction does not lessen the costs which that reproduction imposes on others, nor does it increase the significance of marginal reproductive interests. Of course, questions of the burdens of avoidance do not determine whether the reproductive outcome is desirable or advised, but merely whether a person can be held responsible for undesirable outcomes. It also does not prevent society from acting to prevent the reproduction in question.

Impact on Offspring

Reproduction is said to be irresponsible when it is reasonably foreseeable that the parents will be unable to produce healthy offspring or will otherwise rear them in circumstances that deny them a minimum level of care, nurturing, and protection. Parents who abuse their children by prenatal or postnatal conduct, rear them in disadvantageous circumstances, or pass on genetic or infectious diseases would appear to fit this category.[17] The consequences for offspring, when coupled with an unwillingness or inability to rear and reasonable alternatives to reproduction, would arguably make this reproduction irresponsible.

There is, however, a major problem with finding harm to offspring in these circumstances and hence with claiming that the reproduction is irresponsible. The problem is that the alleged harm to offspring occurs from birth itself. Either the harm is congenital and unavoidable if birth is to occur, or the harm is avoidable after birth occurs, but the parents will not refrain from the harmful action. Preventing harm would mean preventing the birth of the child whose interests one is trying to protect. Yet a child's interests are hardly protected by preventing the child's existence. If the child has no way to be born or raised free of that harm, a person is not injuring the child by enabling her to be born in the circumstances of concern. The overwhelming majority of courts faced with this question in wrongful life cases brought on behalf of the child have reached the same conclusion.[18]

Of course, this objection would not hold if the harmful conditions are such that the very existence of the child, viewed solely in light of his interests as he is then situated, would be a wrong to him. In theory such cases of wrongful life could exist, but it is doubtful whether most of the cases of concern fit that extreme rubric. For example, children born with genetic handicaps or HIV might have years of life that are a good to them, as would children born in illegitimacy, poverty, or to abusive parents, even though it is less good a life than they deserve. In fact, if true cases of wrongful life did arise, one's duty would be to act immediately to prevent continued existence in order to minimize the harm. Protecting offspring by preventing their birth thus does not benefit them, because it denies them the chance to live when existence, despite its limitations, is in their interests.[19]

This point about wrongful life is key to any claim that reproduction is irresponsible because it harms offspring by bringing them into the world in a diseased, handicapped, or disadvantaged condition. If offspring are not injured because there is no alternative way for them to be born absent the condition of concern, then reproduction is not irresponsible because of the effect on offspring who are born less whole than is desirable. This is true both in cases in which the harms are congenitally unavoidable because of genetic or infectious disease and in cases in which the harm is avoidable after birth but the parents will nevertheless injure their offspring. If there is no injury to offspring from their birth alone, then reproduction is not irresponsible because children are born in undesirable circumstances.

Yet one may still condemn giving birth to offspring in such circumstances. Derek Parfit captures this point well in his example of a woman who is told by her physician that if she gets pregnant while on a certain medication she will give birth to a child with a mild deformity, such as a withered arm, but if she waits a month, she can conceive a perfectly normal child.[20] If the woman refuses to wait and has the child with the withered arm, she has not harmed that child, because there is no way that it could have been born normal. Still, many would say that she has acted wrongly because she has gratuitously chosen to bring a suffering child into the world when a brief wait would have enabled her to have a normal, though different, child. Now one could argue that her action is morally justified by the net good provided the child born with the withered arm. However, if one concludes that her actions are wrong, it is not because she has harmed the child born with the withered arm, but because she has violated a norm against offending persons who are troubled by gratuitous suffering.[21]

Burdens on Society

A main ground for charging that reproduction is irresponsible is the cost or burden it imposes on others. This burden may take a financial or nonfinancial form. A common kind of nonfinancial burden is the sense of outrage or offense felt when someone gratuitiously has children who are born with disease or disadvantages, as in Parfit's example of the withered arm. Even though bringing children into the world who have no other practical way to be born healthy does not injure them, it does injure the sensibilities of those persons offended by the action, particularly when the person reproducing could have easily avoided that outcome. In this case, the person reproducing is harming those whose sensibilities are affected by this experience.

But there is a problem in using this notion of offense to condemn those who bring unavoidably handicapped children into the world. The sense of offense is grounded in the undesirability of handicapped or disadvantaged children and is inescapably a judgment about their worth. A claim of irresponsibility that rests on the undesirability of handicapped persons will not be a strong basis for moral condemnation or public action to prevent such births, particularly if those reproducing plan to rear or have other strong reproductive interests in the birth in question and cannot reproduce without risking the handicapped birth.

The most significant burdens on others thus turn out to be the financial costs that reproduction will impose on the public treasury in welfare payments, medical costs, educational costs, child abuse monitoring, social workers, etc. Unspecified costs such as the costs of crime and social disintegration that such reproduction helps cause could also be included here.

Now this category of costs is significant only if it significantly exceeds the costs which any birth imposes on society. It may be that any additional child makes demands on societal resources and incurs public subsidies to some extent. It may also be that only some of those subsidized in this way repay those costs over their lifetime through their own contributions. Only where the costs imposed or the subsidies demanded exceed a reasonable level might one be said to be harming others by their reproduction.

It is difficult to say which cases fall into that category and thus may be deemed irresponsible. Persons who reproduce knowing that they will depend on the welfare system or the charity of others to support their children will be imposing costs on others. The question is, however, whether those costs are beyond what we reasonably expect children to cost and thus are beyond what we are willing to pay to enable persons to have offspring. If the costs do exceed that ceiling, there may be grounds for charging them with irresponsible reproduction because their reproduction requires others to pay more than can be reasonably expected to enable reproduction to occur.

The size of the cost will be determinative when the reproductive interest at stake is small and will be less important as the reproductive interest mounts. Of course, how great that interest must be and how interests compare in individual cases will require close judgments. Such judgments will also affect the validity of state efforts to minimize the costs by discouraging the reproduction.

Another important issue of burdensome and possibly irresponsible reproduction is reproduction in the face of overpopulation. When are additional births irresponsible because of the large number of existing persons? To answer this question, we must first decide how many people there ought to be and then allocate future reproduction accordingly. Parfit has shown that a number based either on the highest possible average level of happiness in the community or the highest total amount of happiness in the community will be inadequate.[22] Such questions raise complex question that are beyond the scope of this book.

Although reproduction may be irresponsible due to overpopulation, this is not the source of the concerns that have led to proposals to use Norplant to prevent irresponsible reproduction in the United States.

The Parameters Applied

With this account of factors relevant to judgments of undesirable or irresponsible reproduction, one can assess the reproductive decisions of particular individuals and groups. The judgment in any given case will reflect a balancing of the reproductive interests at stake, the ease or burdens of avoiding reproduction, and the effects on others. A careful assessment of these factors will often be difficult because of factual uncertainties and normative imponderables about the weight to be assigned to each factor. Yet this is the task that anyone who fairly attempts to judge reproductive responsibility must undertake.

Social Policy Issues

The question whether social policy should discourage irresponsible or undesirable reproduction presents a different set of issues. Even if we agree that reproduction in certain cases is undesirable or irresponsible, the question remains what to do about it. Should reproduction always be left to the individuals involved or are governmental actions to discourage or prevent the reproduction in question appropriate?

Excluding the government as an actor/participant in the dialogue about reproductive responsibility is not justified. The state has responsibilities to protect citizens and to facilitate exercise of their rights. Because reproduction so directly affects others and the state is often called upon to pay the costs of reproduction, there is a legitimate role for the state to speak on these matters.

More controversial, however, are the steps that the state may take to implement its views of reproductive responsibility. These range from providing subsidies, information, education, and access to the use of positive incentives, penalties, and seizures. An important distinction is between governmental programs that support or encourage voluntary choice and those that are more coercive. Programs that inform, educate, assist, and subsidize will be more easily accepted than more coercive actions. However, voluntarism may have dangers, even in purportedly benign government programs. Information can be delivered in settings or in styles that might be perceived as threatening. The very fact that the government is involved constitutes a judgment about the undesirability of conduct and may offends some persons. Charges of genocide or discrimination may arise because a voluntary program appears targeted to a particular ethnic or minority community. In general, however, programs designed to inform women or to provide access to Norplant are desirable and acceptable. This is true even if only particular groups are targeted, such as welfare mothers, teenagers, women with AIDS, or those convicted of child abuse.

More controversial government actions involve programs that offer incentives or condition program benefits in return for certain reproductive choices. In general, incentive programs are designed to preserve autonomy, even though they attempt to influence how the autonomy in question is exercised. However, offering rewards to use Norplant or conditioning the receipt of welfare benefits on its use may be perceived as burdening or coercing individual choice, especially when the choice is presented to welfare mothers, teenagers, and other vulnerable groups. As the discussion below will show, however, the legality of such offers and conditions should be distinguished from their wisdom as social policy. If the incentive offer or condition does not deprive a person of what they are otherwise entitled to, it will usually be legally permissible. However, one can question whether irresponsible reproduction is so serious a problem that focussing on these groups is a sound answer to serious social problems.

More coercive measures, such as penalties for reproducing irresponsibly or refusing birth control, have a strong presumption against them. Prudential questions aside, there may be legal or constitutional barriers against such policies. The power of the state to coerce or force people not to reproduce turns on whether its actions violate a fundamental right, and if so, whether there is a compelling interest to justify it. If the state's action interferes with or limits coital reproduction by a married couple, it would ordinarily be found to infringe upon a fundamental right to procreate and thus require strong justification.[23]

An unresolved question at this point is whether courts evaluating such a claim would assess the importance of the reproduction at issue to the individuals involved. If the parents would rear, mere offense at what they are doing or costs to the taxpayer probably would be insufficient to justify intruding on their right. However, if the parents would not rear, because of unfitness, past neglect, impecunity, or other factors, the courts in particular cases could find that the reproductive interest is so slight as to allow a lesser state interest to justify intrusion.[24] Of course, direct seizures to implant Norplant or to sterilize individuals would require a very strong justification because of the intrusion of bodily integrity.

Policies directed at reproduction by unmarried persons or minors might have a lesser constitutional hurdle to surmount. Because the Supreme Court has not held that persons have a right to reproduce outside marriage, a lesser justification may be needed to uphold such policies.[25] In that case, costs to the community might justify laws that could not be justified against married persons. However, unmarried persons would still have rights against bodily intrusion. Thus state policies that required physical burdens or sacrifice, such as forcible implants or sterilization, would have to meet the compelling interest standard. In those cases saving money or preventing insults to community sensibility may not be sufficient, even if the legally protected reproductive interest is less than in the case of married persons.

It appears that coercive sanctions will be rarely available to states seeking to minimize or discourage irresponsible reproduction. In most instances, the harms sought to be averted are costs to the community or to a sense of offense, because children themselves, who have no way to be born without the disadvantage in question, would not be harmed. These kinds of concerns will not justify coerced intrusions of the body, much less on strong reproductive interests. However, they could justify limitations on lesser reproductive interests, such as genetic reproduction *tout court* or when persons have no protected reproductive interest because of age and marital status. Other than the severely retarded, there may be no group that fits the criteria for coercive action. In the end, government policy will have to rely on information, education, counselling, subsidies, and incentives, so that the freedom of choice in matters of reproduction is protected.

Five Problematic Cases

With the parameters of reproductive responsibility and the range of policy options as background, we are now ready to discuss five problematic situations for which Norplant has been urged. In each case, we must balance the benefits of the questionable reproduction to the person involved against the claims of irresponsibility. The availability of state policies to discourage undesirable reproduction will depend upon the extent to which those policies that interfere with fundamental rights can be justified by harmful effects on offspring, taxpayers, and society. The discussion will show that in most instances the alleged irresponsibility will not support coercive policies, though it will permit voluntary measures that use education, information, subsidies, and incentives.

1. Contraception As a Condition of Probation

The question of compulsory use of Norplant has been most frequently raised in cases involving women convicted of child abuse or homicide of their children. In these cases, the sentencing judge is faced with a problem. Although a prison sentence is justified, the judge recognizes that the woman might be better rehabilitated in the community. However, she also knows that if the woman has more children, rehabilitation will be more difficult and that there is a real danger that the abuse of the new child might occur. In these situations, some judges have offered women the option of probation on the condition that they consent to Norplant or other contraception as an alternative to the prison sentence that would otherwise be imposed.[26]

The most widely publicized case of mandatory contraception, *People v. Johnson,* involved a twenty-seven-year-old woman sentenced to two to four years in prison for child abuse.[27] She had been convicted of severely beating two of her four children with a belt. Toward the end of her first year, the trial judge offered to release the woman on probation if she would agree to have Norplant implanted for three years of probation. The woman initially agreed. Later she sought to appeal this sentence on the ground that it was coerced, that it violated her fundamental right to procreate, and that it was medically contraindicated.

In a rehearing after the woman revoked her initial agreement to the sentence, the judge noted that she had shown herself incapable of caring for her children and stated:

> . . . It is in the defendant's best interest and certainly in any unconceived child's interest that she not have any more children until she is mentally and emotionally prepared to do so. The birth of additional children until after she has successfully completed the court-ordered mental health counseling and parenting classes dooms both her and any subsequent children to repeat this vicious cycle.[28]

He further noted:

> Although the right to procreate is substantial and constitutionally protected, it is not absolute and can be limited in a proper case. The compelling state interest in the protection of the children supersedes this particular individual's right to procreate and does not interfere with her right of sexual expression.[29]

In considering the validity of contraception as a condition of probation, an important preliminary issue is whether the judge's sentencing power includes the power to impose contraception as a condition of probation. If the law does not authorize such a sentence, then such conditions are invalid.[30] If such probation conditions have been authorized, the question then is whether the authorized sentence is unconstitutional.

Ordinarily a state requirement or coercive offer that a woman take Norplant would require a compelling justification, for it intrudes into her body and limits her reproduction. A convicted child abuser could still have an interest in reproducing. She may wish to have and rear more children, precisely because of guilt she feels for her past behavior. However, if she will lose custody of any child upon birth because of her past record as an abuser, her reproductive interest may be reduced. If custody will not automatically be removed, or if she will be permitted to have some limited contact with offspring, her reproductive interest increases in importance. Even if she has no rearing role, she may still get satisfaction from having produced another child. Although the facts of individual cases will vary, convicted child abusers will often retain the reproductive interests that enjoy presumptive protected status.

If that is so, any coercive state efforts to prevent her from reproduction would have to meet the compelling interest test. In this case the asserted state interest, protection of offspring who will be injured by future abuse, will not necessarily occur. If the woman retains custody, she may have been rehabilitated and no longer be an abuser. Social workers may more closely monitor her to prevent abuse from occurring.[31] Even if she does abuse future children, it is not clear that they will enjoy such a horrible life that they never should have been born at all and thus are harmed by being born to an abusing mother.[32] In short, the need to protect future offspring does not appear to justify overriding her right to procreate because the means of protection prevents the birth of the children whom one is trying to protect.

Nor could limitations on her reproduction be justified by the need to protect society and the community. Child abusers who reproduce will cost the community more money and services in monitoring, treatment, and other services. If children are born and later injured, many people will experience outrage at her repetitive conduct. More demand on scarce foster parent resources will occur at a time when those resources are severely strained. Costly medical and psychological treatment may be needed for the child.[33] In addition, people may lose confidence in a system that permits a woman who has severely beaten or murdered her children to produce more children. But these costs would not ordinarily support coercive sanctions that limit exercise of a fundamental right and probably would not support coercive sanctions for failure to use Norplant.

However, the woman in question is a convicted child abuser and could be sent to prison. A condition of imprisonment is that men and women are ordinarily prevented from reproducing—from begetting and bearing children while in prison.[34] They have no constitutional right to conjugal visits, and no right to hand their sperm out for artificial insemination.[35] Since prisoners are ordinarily deprived of procreation during the term of imprisonment, could not the state place a person subject to imprisonment on probation with contraception on the ground that the greater power to imprison implies the lesser power to impose contraception?

If the greater power to imprison does not imply the lesser power to impose contraception, then interfering in reproduction in this way will be a punishment that must satisfy Eighth Amendment standards against cruel and unusual punishment.[36] This provision bars punishments that are excessive or barbarous.[37] Because temporary loss of reproduction via Norplant does not appear to be excessive for the crime of abusing children, the question will turn on whether imposition of Norplant is inherently cruel or barbarous. Here the method is a choice—probation with Norplant or prison—that is akin to the choices presented to defendants deciding whether to plead guilty, but one that focuses on their body and its functions. It causes them to accept a minor surgical intervention into their body, some side effects of varying intensity, and the loss of procreative ability for a period of time.

One cannot predict with certainty how courts would rule on a claim that such a punishment violates the Eighth Amendment. Bodily and reproductive intrusions are clearly not favored, yet Norplant is not so highly intrusive or shocking, given the restrictions that usually occur with imprisonment, that offering the persons a choice that will temporarily limit their reproductive ability for a period of time as punishment for crime would necessarily be found to be unconstitutional. However, the question is a close one and cannot be decided without more particular facts. Because the restriction is rationally related to rehabilitation and to preventing the very crimes being punished, the ultimate decision will hinge on perceptions of the need for the state to mandate reproductive restrictions.[38]

In sum, the validity of compulsory contraception for convicted child abusers depends on whether the limitation of procreation must be independently justified or is a rational, nonbarbarous punishment for serious crime. If the former, the state justifications are insufficient. Neither the interest in protecting unborn offspring from harm nor in saving social welfare resources justifies limiting procreation. Only if persons subject to imprisonment but placed on probation have fewer procreative rights would such a condition of probation be acceptable. Even then, one can question whether a technological solution to the problem should be sought.

2. Compulsory Contraception to Prevent Congenital Disease

The case for compulsory contraception to prevent the birth of offspring with congenital disease is also hard to sustain. One target of such efforts would be couples who are at risk for having children with genetic handicaps and yet insist on reproducing. Ordinarily, they would have a one in two or one in four chance of having a child with the defect in question. Depending on the disease, the child could die early or have a lifetime of chronic illness and medical care. However, this is a relatively small group whose overall numbers do not justify such an intrusive intervention.

A more likely target would be women who are HIV positive. They have a 25 to 35% chance of passing HIV on to their offspring.[39] If they do, the child may die early or be maintained at high cost for many years. Even if children are not infected, the parents still are at risk of dying and leaving their children parentless. Indeed, the problem of children who are parentless due to AIDS is a growing social problem, with 80,000 such children predicted by the year 2000.[40]

In either case, however, the compulsory use of Norplant cannot be justified. To begin with, members of both groups have substantial interests in reproduction. The couple that has had a handicapped child may hope for a healthy child, but be willing to raise and care for another child with the handicap in question. Moreover, the risk of a child with handicap will ordinarily be one in four, or perhaps one in two. Preventing the birth of the handicapped child would also prevent the greater likelihood that offspring will not have the disease in question. Avoiding the birth of an affected child may also require prenatal testing and abortion to which the parents are opposed.

Similarly, women with HIV may still find procreation immensely meaningful, both because it is a prime source of meaning and validation in their social-cultural context and because it meets their need for continuity after the death looming over them. As Nancy Dubler and Carol Levine note, in the view of these women

> having babies . . . may be the most reasonable and available choice, a natural outcome of all the the forces in their lives, in which avenues for self-definition and expression other than mothering are largely absent.[41]

Even if particular individuals will not rear affected offspring or will not rear for long, core interests of reproduction are at stake for both groups.

The case for claiming that their reproduction is irresponsible must therefore rest on the burdens which it imposes on offspring and society. The burden commonly cited is that they are knowingly having or risking having children who are born with serious genetic or infectious diseases. The children who are born with HIV may face an early death or a period of health and normal growth until symptoms arise. They will then face repeated hospitalizations and an early death. If they do not themselves have HIV, they are likely to be born into circumstances in which their parents will soon die, and they may end up in foster care or other disadvantageous circumstances.

Similarly, children born with serious genetic handicaps may face repeated surgeries and hospitalizations, significant mortality and morbidity, social stigma, and the suffering that arises from their mental and physical limitations. While their parents may rear them, some of them will be placed in poorly funded state institutions or group homes.

Yet in both cases one cannot say that these children have been harmed by being born, because they have no way to be born free of the congenital diseases or social circumstances that are so disadvantageous.[42] Unlike Parfit's case of the risk of a withered arm, the persons procreating here cannot produce a healthy child by postponing conception. All their offspring are at risk for the conditions of concern. Few of those conditions would make the child's life so horrible that their interests would have been best served by never being born.[43] Thus it is unlikely that the goal of preventing harm to offspring by preventing them from being born would justify a coercive contraceptive policy toward their parents.

Nor will the significant costs that they may impose on the public treasury and charity justify such a policy. In some instances the parents will not impose rearing costs on others, because they will bear the cost themselves, either directly or through insurance. However, in most cases the persons reproducing with this risk will end up requiring large subsidies from the state for medical care and other services for their children. If the children's diseases are serious enough, as AIDS and some genetic conditions are, they will be demanding subsidies greater than those ordinarily provided to person who reproduce. In addition, there may be other social costs, from the degradation of many orphans in impoverished settings to the offense felt at the actions of persons who do not attempt to avoid reproduction when the risks of an abnormal birth are great.

None of these costs, however, are sufficient to justify directly imposing Norplant or other contraception on women at risk for offspring with these conditions. Because their reproductive interest is generally a strong one, only very compelling needs would justify overriding their fundamental right to procreate. Saving money and preventing offense ordinarily would not rise to the required level. However, a closer analysis of their reproductive interest could on occasion yield a different conclusion. For example, if they lack the capacity or interest in rearing, plan to institutionalize the child at birth, or face a short life span due to their own illness, required contraception would not violate more significant a reproductive interest than if they intended to rear for long periods.[44] Because the bodily intrusion may be relatively minor, it may be that compelled contraception in rare cases could be justified, though such policies would be highly controversial.

At present this discussion is largely hypothetical, however, because no one has proposed that women infected with HIV or those at genetic risk should be penalized for reproduction or failure to accept Norplant. These remedies seem so extreme because of the seriousness of the intrusion and the lack of sufficient justification for it. They would also be open to charges of racism and discrimination against those who are less than able-bodied.

The more immediate policy question concerns the lengths to which the state may go to persuade these groups voluntarily to avoid reproduction. In both cases the state could support or conduct programs to make sure that persons at risk are aware of the potential consequences of their reproductive behavior and that contraception and abortion to avert reproduction is available. Included in such information would be facts concerning prenatal or other tests to inform them of their risk status or the status of a fetus.[45]

Much more controversial is whether the state or private parties should engage in directive counselling, urging that they not reproduce because of the risks of affected offspring and the other problems thereby caused. Health care providers, counsellors, and ethicists are currently split over whether directed counselling can be justified in these cases.[46] This debate is largely prudential rather than ethical. As long as directed counselling leaves the woman free to make her own choice, it would not violate her autonomy. Indeed, it may be useful to make her aware of the serious consequences of her actions. However, any mandatory or directive program will be controversial whatever its ethical or policy justification because of the perception that it is singling out women who are already stigmatized, and because of the risk that it denigrates the worth of the children whose birth it is trying to avoid.

3. Welfare Issues

Compulsory contraception through Norplant has also emerged as an issue of welfare policy. Shortly after the FDA approved Norplant, legislators in Kansas, Oklahoma, and Louisiana introduced bills offering financial rewards to welfare mothers who agreed to Norplant implants. The rewards ranged from $100 in Louisiana to $500 in Kansas, with Kansas also offering a yearly maintenance fee of $50. Welfare would also pay the costs of the Norplant. Similar proposals are likely in other states.

Although none of these proposals has passed, the appeal of Norplant as a way to control costly reproduction by poor women is obvious. A common perception is that high welfare costs are the result of poor women having children to cash in on welfare benefits. The editorial board of the *Philadelphia Inquirer* fell prey to this myth when, in an editorial entitled "Norplant and the Underclass," it praised Norplant as an answer to problems of welfare associated with a high minority birth rate (when the black community protested, the newspaper quickly apologized).[47] A common sentiment is that poor women are acting irresponsibly when they have children that the taxpayers will have to support. If so, the idea of encouraging them to use contraception makes sense.

But is reproduction when one will require public assistance to support offspring irresponsible? A person who intends to rear such offspring, as most welfare mothers do, will have a significant reproductive interest at stake. However, to realize their reproductive goal they will be demanding that the community pay rearing costs that those who reproduce are usually responsible for. Is it unreasonable to ask the community to do so? A good argument can be made that it is, particularly if one has already reproduced and could do so at some point in the future. Only if there are no reproductive alternatives for that person or if avoidance is not reasonably possible might that action be reasonable.

Yet even if a mild judgment of irresponsibility can be lodged, it would not follow that compulsory contraceptive measures are justified. Indeed, as a legal matter, the state probably could not penalize persons for giving birth to children who need welfare, even if moral culpability could be shown. The injury to the community's resources and norms of proper reproduction is simply insufficient to justify coercive intrusion upon a fundamental right. Nor have such proposals been seriously made.

Instead, the focus of policy has been on proposals to encourage women on welfare to use Norplant voluntarily. While no one objects to informing welfare mothers of the Norplant option and providing it free of charge, proposals to pay women to have the implant or to require it as a condition of receiving welfare are more controversial. Neither idea unconstitutionally infringes upon procreative liberty. However, one may question whether the costs of excessive births by welfare mothers are such a serious problem that direct state intervention in reproductive decisions is advisable.

Paying Rewards   The idea of paying a reward, whether $100, $500, or some higher sum, to accept and maintain Norplant does not violate procreative liberty. In trying to influence or manage reproductive choice, the reward assumes that such choice exists. Although $100 may be attractive enough to get a woman's attention, it does not deny her something that she would otherwise receive and thus should not be considered coercive. A woman remains free to reject the implant, even though she will not receive the reward or the other benefits of long-lasting, convenient contraception. The idea of manipulating incentives to reduce reproduction is no more offensive than the manipulation of incentives to get welfare mothers to work or marry. No one has proposed so high a sum (say, over $1000) that a charge of exploitation or coercion is more credible.

Still, rewards for using Norplant will remain controversial, with groups supportive of welfare rights and procreative choice split on its acceptability. For example, some affiliates of Planned Parenthood of America, a main defender of reproductive choice, have conducted experiments paying teenage mothers a per diem stipend to avoid further pregnancy.[48] Such a policy would implicitly support rewards for accepting Norplant.

Many other liberal groups oppose payments to avoid reproduction, arguing that any reward to impoverished persons is coercive.[49] Even if a \$100 or \$500 reward is not coercive, it implicitly denigrates welfare mothers by assuming that they cannot rationally weigh the pros and cons of reproduction without the enticement of a reward. Also, such a program has the appearance of bartering their reproductive potential for money, a practice not acceptable with organ donations. It puts the state in the position of buying their right to have children and thus paying to avoid poor and minority births.

The question of paying welfare mothers to accept Norplant is less legal or ethical and more a question of symbols and appearances. Given the symbolic connotations associated with bribing welfare mothers not to reproduce, the preferred strategy is education, counselling about the merits of Norplant, and ensuring access to all welfare mothers who want it. A concentrated educational campaign might reach most of the target group without incurring the symbolic costs of buying up their right to reproduce. Only if few women respond to that option should a reward system for Norplant be implemented. However, since such rewards can be respectful of reproductive choice, they should not automatically be foreclosed.

As a Condition of Welfare   Even more questionable would be a policy that made acceptance of Norplant a condition of receiving welfare payments at all. Proposals linking welfare to sterilization surfaced repeatedly in the 1960s and 1970s, but never gained much support. Norplant, however, is less intrusive than sterilization and completely reversible. With renewed interest in tying welfare to job training, job seeking, number of children, and even marriage, it would not be surprising if some states require acceptance of Norplant as a condition of receiving welfare payments.[50]

Legally, such a condition probably would be constitutional. Since a state has no constitutional obligation to provide welfare at all, it would be free to provide it only if certain conditions rationally related to the program are met.[51] A condition relating to contraception that would enable recipients to take care of current children and lower costs might be found rational in a welfare system that is attempting to reduce costs and help women into the job market. It is clearly distinguishable from unconstitutional welfare conditions that condition benefits on the exercise or waiver of constitutional rights that are unrelated to the purposes of a welfare system, such as one's political party, one's religious affiliation, or the books one chooses to read.[52]

Legality aside, however, one can question whether any state should go so far. Simply making Norplant available will lead many women on welfare to choose it. A limited reward system would increase those numbers. Making Norplant a condition of receiving welfare seems too strenuous an intervention in reproductive choice. It will also penalize dependent children whose living standard decreases because of their mother's unwillingness to have the implant. Given available alternatives, the case for conditioning any welfare payment on Norplant is not a strong one.

4. Compulsory Contraception for the Retarded

Controlling the reproduction of mentally retarded persons has a checkered history in the United States. In the early twentieth century the American Eugenics Society actively lobbied to sterilize "mental defectives" and "feeble-minded persons" because of a perceived threat to the gene pool and social welfare. The result was compulsory sterilization laws passed in over thirty states which the United States Supreme Court upheld in 1927 in *Buck v. Bell*.[53] With this imprimatur, more than 60,000 persons were sterilized over the next thirty years.

In the 1960s a strong reaction to compulsory eugenic sterilization occurred, impelled by awareness of the excesses of Nazi eugenic practices and the scientific unsoundness of the hereditary assumptions underlying these laws. It also became clear that many persons had been sterilized who were neither mentally ill nor retarded, including Carrie Buck, the original plaintiff in *Buck v. Bell*.[54] Although that case has never been reversed, compulsory sterilization is now generally viewed as a gross violation of human rights and no longer performed for eugenic reasons.

In the mid-1970s, however, it became clear that there were some circumstances in which sterilization was justified to protect the retarded from pregnancy rather than to serve eugenics or save money. For example, retarded women in state institutions or group homes are vulnerable to sexual exploitation or rape. Pregnancy, especially in women who lack comprehension, poses serious health risks. Delivery by Caesarean section may be necessary. Often parents restrict participation in group homes and other opportunities to avoid having their retarded daughters risk pregnancy.

Faced with parents seeking to have retarded daughters sterilized, state courts began authorizing such procedures. Since few states still had statutes authorizing such sterilizations, the main issue before the courts was whether a probate court's inherent *parens patriae* power over incompetent patients authorized them to order sterilization in the absence of statutory authority when it seemed in the incompetent ward's interest.[55] While some courts preferred to wait for legislative authorization, influential state supreme courts, including those of New Jersey, Massachusetts, and Washington, devised tests that allowed sterilization when it could be shown to benefit the incompetent ward.[56]

Norplant presents an attractive alternative in situations in which sterilization would otherwise be appropriate. Because there is usually no serious reproductive interest at stake, the main question is whether implantation of Norplant will cause harm. If sterilization is justified, *a fortiori* Norplant should be because it is less intrusive and reversible. Indeed, it would seem preferable to sterilization. Thus parents or guardians who petition for sterilization should show that less restrictive contraceptive measures such as Norplant are contraindicated or not available.

In fact, it may be acceptable for parents or caretakers to have Norplant routinely implanted in mentally retarded and institutionalized women concerned about their risk of pregnancy. Because surgical insertion is required, the consent of parents or guardians is necessary, though the judicial review required for sterilization should not be. Norplant may thus provide a technological solution to the risk of pregnancy faced by mentally retarded women.

Controlling reproduction in severely retarded women with Norplant limits procreation without limiting procreative choice, for the notion of reproductive choice is no more meaningful for severely retarded women than is electoral choice. If they are so mentally impaired that the concept of reproduction and parenthood has no meaning, then limiting their reproduction does not infringe upon their procreative liberty. The concept of procreative choice simply does not apply to them.[57] If mistakes are made about reproductive interest, the Norplant can simply be removed.

Of course, the retarded do have rights of bodily integrity and the right to be treated with respect. They should not be burdened merely to serve the needs of others. Limiting their reproduction, however, does not harm them and actually serves their interests by protecting them from the physical risks of pregnancy. If done with a minimum of bodily intrusion, as occurs with Norplant, such limits should be socially acceptable as well. However, careful monitoring of how Norplant is used with this population, including indications, side effects, and length of use, is needed before implantation can routinely occur. With these protections, the use of Norplant with the retarded at the request of parents and guardians may be acceptable.

5. Norplant and Adolescents

Norplant has also been suggested as an answer to teenage pregnancy. If informed consent is obtained, the use of Norplant poses no issues beyond those raised by teenage contraceptive use generally. The chief issue here is whether teenagers can obtain contraceptives without parental consent or notification. If state law permits adolescent females to obtain medically prescribed contraceptives, then they should be able to obtain Norplant as well.

Also, there should be no barrier to parents or guardians providing Norplant to adolescent girls who desire it. The discretionary power of parents to rear their children entitles them to obtain medical care that is in their child's interests. Postponing pregnancy until a more mature time serves the interests of child and parent. While parents should not be able to have doctors insert Norplant against a teenager's wishes, there should be no objection if the child agrees with the parent's desire for Norplant.

Programs that offer Norplant in school clinics are more controversial, however, because the state appears to be taking a more active role in controlling adolescent reproduction. The Baltimore school system, which now provides Norplant along with other contraceptives, has been careful to preserve choice in offering Norplant to a teenage population with an exceedingly high pregnancy rate.[58] The young women are informed of the risks and benefits of the implant and are not pressured in any way to accept it. Parents are notified if the teenager consents to their being notified. However, some people are troubled by the idea of city authorities trying to influence female reproduction and doubt whether such programs are truly noncoercive.

A more hypothetical question is whether the state could require that teenage girls have an antifertility vaccine or Norplant implantation shortly after puberty, after one illegitimate birth, or some other risk marker in order to make pregnancy a matter of deliberate choice.[59] This policy would prevent teenage pregnancy, but would not prevent girls who wish to have children from regaining fertility by having the implants removed or the vaccine rendered inactive.

Given the very high rates of unintended teenage pregnancy, such a policy would no doubt have many supporters. And would it not necessarily violate the procreative liberty of its targets, for it only temporarily postpones pregnancy and is aimed at unmarried adolescents who do not have the same right to reproduce that adults do. If the intrusion is viewed as minor,[60] they will have ample time to have and rear children when they decide to do so. Such a policy would prevent many illegitimate births and the cycle of dropping out of high school, poor employment opportunities, and welfare that adolescent pregnancy often brings. Also, it would prevent the birth of children who themselves are often doomed to repeat that cycle or who grow up without male authority figures in their life. Although such children are not wronged by being born, society may still prefer that children be born with more advantages.

Although the purpose is commendable and teenagers may lack a right to reproduce, a policy of compulsory contraception will face high constitutional barriers. Teenagers do have a strong interest in bodily integrity. The insertion of the device may be viewed as minor, but the the potential side effects are serious enough—many women cannot tolerate Norplant—to make the bodily intrusion substantial. Overriding this interest may be difficult to justify despite the worthiness of the goal.

A further problem would arise in identifying the target of such an intrusive policy. If directed at all female adolescents, it would be grossly broad, intruding upon the many to prevent pregnancy by a few.[61] If targeted to subgroups that have high rates of pregnancy, it risks actual or perceived discrimination on racial or ethnic grounds. In its most defensible form, it would apply only to teenagers who already had a teenage pregnancy and refused to use contraception. Yet even there the intrusiveness of forcing a contraceptive implant on an unwilling subject would be a difficult barrier to overcome.

In short, such an intrusive policy of social engineering sounds too Orwellian to be acceptable, even if the state possessed the raw constitutional power to implement it. As with most instances of allegedly irresponsible reproduction, it is far preferable to rely on education and choice rather than on mandatory measures. Indeed, a fair attempt to encourage contraceptive use by adolescents would probably obviate the need for involuntary implantation.

Conclusion

Procreation is a basic right, but it is not an absolute right. Its protected status does not relieve individuals of the moral obligation to reproduce responsibly. When they do not, public pressure arises to use reversible technologies such as Norplant to limit their reproduction.

Unless voluntarily chosen, however, the use of Norplant or other contraceptives can rarely be justified as a solution to problems of allegedly irresponsible reproduction. Its most defensible application is with severely retarded females who are at risk of sexual exploitation or rape. In the other situations discussed, however, its intrusiveness and effect on procreation make it highly suspect. Child abusers, women infected with HIV, welfare mothers, and teenagers have interests in procreation or bodily integrity which mandatory use of Norplant violates. Neither protection of future offspring nor conservation of public funds are compelling enough reasons to justify intrusions on such basic rights. In addition, there is the danger of discrimination or antipathy toward targeted groups.

This conclusion should not prevent the state from informing women of the Norplant option, subsidizing its provision, or even offering financial incentives to use it. If these alternatives are pursued, the need for compulsory contraception through Norplant further weakens. Forcible limitations on reproduction need a much stronger justification than these cases present.

NOTES

1. Norplant illustrates well the themes of autonomy and ambivalence that pervade this book. The ambivalence is strong because it involves the state in mandating particular reproductive outcomes. Even if justified in particular circumstances, state involvement sets a dangerous precedent that could lead to less compelling instances of forced contraception.

2. This approval culminated twenty years of research and development sponsored by the Population Council and made available to American women a contraceptive that since 1966 has been used by more than 55,000 women in forty-six countries.

3. The drug is contained in the silastic capsules in dry, crystalline form. Stacey Arthur, "The Norplant Prescription: Birth Control, Woman Control or Crime Control," *UCLA Law Review*, 40 (1993): 1.

4. P. D. Darney et al., "Acceptance and Perceptions of Norplant Among Users in San Francisco, USA," *Studies in Family Planning* 21 (1990): 152; D. Shoupe et al., "The Signficance of Bleeding Patterns in Norplant Users," *Obstetrics and Gynecology* 77 (1991): 256.

5. Easy removal assumes that a physician is available and willing to do the procedure. Finding a physician to remove Norplant is a problem in some Third World settings and in situations in which the physician disagrees with the woman's decision to stop the contraceptive. There may also be a cost barrier to removal.

6. Norplant, like other contraceptives, is not usually covered by health insurance policies. Tamar Lewin, "Wide Use Seen For an Implant in Birth Control," *New York Times*, 29 November 1991.

7. Other contraceptives, such as Depo-Provera—which lasts three months—and Orvil, the "morning after pill," should also be made available.

8. State of Washington, 52nd Leg., reg. sess., H.R. 2909.

9. Editorial, "Poverty and Norplant: Can Contraception Reduce the Underclass?," *Philadelphia Inquirer*, 12 December 1990. A vehement protest from black journalists and the black community led to an apology. "Apology: The Editorial on 'Norplant and Poverty' Was Misguided and Wrongheaded," *Philadelphia Inquirer*, 23 December 1990.

10. "Governor's Welfare Plan Pushes Free Birth Control," *New York Times*, 17 January 1993.

11. Tamar Lewin, "Baltimore School Clinics to Offer Birth Control by Surgical Implant," *New York Times*, 4 December 1992.

12. Matthew Rees, "Shot in the Arm," *The New Republic*, 9 December 1991.

13. There is more willingness to impose limitations on noncoital reproduction, usually because its connection with the freedom to procreate is not recognized. See chapters 2, 5, and 6.

14. Phillip Reilly, *The Surgical Solution* (Baltimore: Johns Hopkins University Press, 1991).

15. *Relf v. Weinberger,* 386 F. Supp. 1384 (D.C. D.Ct. 1974). As a result of the Relf litigation, informed consent and a thirty-day waiting period are now required for sterilization in federally funded programs. Note, "Coerced Sterilization Under Federally Funded Family Planning Programs," *New England Law Review* 11 (1976): 589–614. See also Reilly, 150–52.

16. One could also talk about the reproductive responsibility of society—its obligation to make sure that safe and healthy means of reproduction or its avoidance are available, including resources that children brought into the world need in order to have a healthy and productive life.

17. Here we must distinguish between unavoidable prenatal harm and prenatal or postnatal harm that is avoidable, but which cannot be avoided under the circumstances. See Chapter 8.

18. See *Smith v. Cote,* 128 N.H. 231, 513 A.2d 341 (1986); *Becker v. Schwartz,* 46 N.Y.2d 401, 386 N.E.2d 807, 413 N.Y.S.2d 895 (1978); *Nelson v. Krusen,* 678 S.W.2d 918 (1984).

19. Of course, there is no guarantee that the remedial action mitigating against the harm will occur.

20. Derek Parfit, "On Doing the Best for Our Children," in *Ethics and Population*, ed. M.D. Bayles (Cambridge, Mass.: Schenkman, 1976).

21. In this example—unlike most of the situations discussed in this chapter— the woman has an alternative way to have a healthy child. She can simply wait a month.

22. Derek Parfit, *Reason and Persons* (New York: Oxford University Press, 1984); David Heyd, *Genethics: The Moral Issues in the Creation of People* (Berkeley: University of California Press, 1992).

23. Although not enumerated in the text of the Constitution, such a belief doubtlessly has constitutional status. Reproduction is so basic to human life and meaning that deprivation without consent would be widely acknowledged as a violation of a fundamental liberty. Indeed, the Supreme Court has acknowledged the existence of such a right in dicta in several cases. See chapter 2.

24. The relevance of whether they have reproduced already or could reproduce in the future under more felicitous circumstances is unclear.

25. See discussion of this point in chapter 2. Note that the issue is whether unmarried persons have the right to engage in coitus or have access to noncoital means of reproduction such as IVF. Once conception occurs, they clearly have a right to go to term, and once birth occurs, to rear offspring. But it does not follow that they have a right to conceive in the first place, even though they cannot be denied the right to gestate a formed fetus or rear a born child.

26. Because Norplant is easily monitored and requires a one-time intervention, it is preferable to a general condition to use birth control or to avoid pregnancy.

27. Tamar Lewin, "Implanted Birth Control Device Renews Debate Over Forced Contraception," *New York Times*, 10 January 1991.

28. Michael Lev, "Judge Firm on Forced Contraception," *New York Times*, 11 January 1991.

29. See Stacey Arthur, "The Norplant Prescription."

30. At least one court has struck down such a condition on this ground. See Stacey Arthur, "The Norplant Prescription."

31. A major limitation with this point, however, is that most child welfare agencies are so overworked and underfunded that they may not be reliable monitors of the offender's behavior with future children. Also, adequate foster care to protect the children may not be available. The less restrictive alternative of monitoring and removal to foster care may be more a theoretical than a real protection of future children from convicted child abusers.

32. The claim that contraception is justified to protect unborn offspring has cogency only if the offspring would have a life so burdened with suffering that it would not be worth living. But even serious child abuse does not appear to cause a life of such unremitting suffering that the child's life is wrongful—i.e., that the child would have preferred no life at all and would commit suicide at the first available opportunity. For example, from the perspective of the child, even a life being abused by parents would seem preferable to no life at all.

33. For example, offspring of cocaine-addicted women cost the medical care system many times what other babies do.

34. Of course, if the woman is pregnant when she enters prison or manages to get pregnant while in there, she cannot be forced or prevented from having an abortion. However, conjugal visits are not constitutionally required, and an inmate has no right to hand his wife sperm for use in artificial insemination outside prison.

35. *Goodwin v. Turner*, 908 F.2d 1395 (8th Cir. 1990).

36. It may be that loss of the greater power to imprison and to prevent reproduction while in prison is based on an essential feature of prison administration and is not an inherent or necessary part of punishment.

37. *Gregg v. Georgia*, 428 U.S. 153 (1976); *Rummel v. Estelle*, 445 U.S. 263 (1980).

38. If Norplant as a condition of probation surmounted previous hurdles, it would still face equal protection problems. All of the mandatory contraception cases to date have involved women, even though men are also convicted of child abuse. Perhaps this is because women are more likely to care for children and thus are more likely to be in a position to repeat their abusive behavior. But men sentenced to prison for child abuse could claim a violation of equal protection if they are not given the same option of temporary contraception that women are. This challenge would be especially powerful if both husband and wife were convicted of child abuse and the woman was offered the option of Norplant while the husband was sent to prison.

39. John Arras, "AIDS and Reproductive Decisions: Having Children in Fear and Trembling," *The Milbank Quarterly* 68, no. 3 (1990): 353, 367.

40. David Michaels and Carol Levine, "Estimates of the Number of Motherless Youth Orphaned by AIDS in the United States," *Journal of the American Medical Association* 268, no. 24 (1992): 3456. The authors argue that ignoring this problem "invites a social catastrophe of the greatest magnitude" because the "death of a parent . . . is one of the most traumatic experiences any child can suffer. When that death is accompanied by stigma and isolation and is followed by instability and insecurity, as it is in AIDS, the potential for trouble, both immediately and in the future is magnified." Id., 3460.

41. C. Levine and N. Dubler, "Uncertain Risks and Bitter Realities: The Reproductive Choices of HIV-Infected Women," *Milbank Quarterly* 68, no. 3 (1990): 321, 323. For women trapped by poverty, illness, crime, and other humiliations, "[a] baby is the chance to have something concrete to love, or, as important, to be loved by. It is proof of fertility and the visible sign of having been loved or at least touched by another." Id., 334. The importance of reproducing is even greater if the woman will die of her disease because of her need to "leave someone behind for a mother or husband to care for in the future . . . the link to immortality that genealogy presents. Id., 335.

42. This case may be contrasted with the Bladerunner problem in chapter 7, where the procreator could make offspring healthy and whole but chooses, out of perverse malice or narcissism, to make the child worse than she need be.

43. The strongest case for such a claim might be Tay-Sachs disease, but that disease would also present a strong case for nontreatment early in the onset of the disease so that any harm to the child from mere existence could be mitigated.

44. Such persons may still have a substantial interest in reproducing. For example, women infected with HIV who will die in a short time may still find great meaning in having a child whom they will not rear for long. See Dubler and Levine.

45. While the state could require that providers inform at-risk persons of the availability of such tests, it is less clear whether the state could require such testing to occur. It may be that minimally intrusive tests that leave the person free to act on the results would not interfere with procreative choice and would serve a useful function. By contrast, requiring known carriers of genetic disease to use birth control or to abort affected fetuses would clearly interfere with procreative liberty.

46. John Arras, "AIDS and Reproductive Decisions: Having Children in Fear and Trembling," *The Milbank Quarterly* 68, no. 3 (1990): 353.

47. "Apology: The Editorial on 'Norplant and Poverty' Was Misguided and Wrongheaded," *Philadelphia Inquirer*, 23 December 1990.

48. Nancy Kates, *Buying Time: The Dollar-a-Day Program* (case study written at the request of Professor Marc Roberts for use at the Kennedy School of Government,

Harvard University, 1990). See also Lucy Williams, "The Ideology of Division: Behavior Modification Welfare Reform Proposals," *Yale Law Journal* 102 (1992): 719, 737.

49. The philosophical literature on coercion is complex and would only rarely find that an offer of a benefit to which the person is not otherwise entitled is coercive. However, see David Zimmerman, "Coercive Wage Offers," *Philosophy and Public Affairs* 10 (1981): 121.

50. Note here the Wisconsin and New Jersey plans and other attempts to get people off of welfare by such conditions. See Isabel Wilkerson, "Wisconsin Welfare Plan: To Reward the Married," *New York Times*, 2 February 1991.

51. *Maher v. Roe,* 432 U.S. 464 (1977); *Harris v. McCrae,* 448 U.S. 297 (1980); *Dandridge v. Williams,* 397 U.S. 471 (1970).

52. Kathleen Sullivan, "Unconstitutional Constitutions," *Harvard Law Review* 102 (1989): 1413.

53. *Buck v. Bell,* 274 U.S. 200 (1927).

54. Paul A. Lombardo, "Three Generations, No Imbeciles: New Light on *Buck v. Bell,*" *New York University Law Review* 60 (1985): 30. This is an insightful and intriguing historical analysis of the deficiencies in the factual basis of that decision.

55. *In re Guardianship of Eberhardy,* 102 Wis.2d 539, 307 N.W.2d 881 (1981).

56. See, e.g., *In re Grady,* 85 N.J. 235, 426 A.2d 467 (1981); *In re Moe,* 385 Mass. 555, 432 N.E.2d 712 (1982); *In re Guardianship of Hayes,* 93 Wash.2d 228, 608 P.2d 635 (1980).

57. This argument is developed in Robertson, "Procreative Liberty and the Control of Conception, Pregnancy, and Childbirth," *Virginia Law Review* 69 (1983): 405, 411–13.

58. Tamar Lewin, "Baltimore School Clinics to Offer Birth Control by Surgical Implant," *New York Times*, 4 December 1992.

59. An antifertility vaccine has not yet been developed, though is an important area of future research. To be acceptable, it would also have to have a limited duration of efficacy and be reversible when one wished to restore fertility. See Carl Dejerassi, "The Bitter Pill," *Science* 245 (1989): 356, 359.

60. One may disagree with this assessment, particularly because of the side effects that many young women would experience.

61. Even though there is a high rate of teenage pregnancy, only a very small percentage of female adolescents become pregnant.

John D. Arras and Jeffrey Blustein

Reproductive Responsibility and Long-Term Contraceptives

In the "good old days" prior to the advent of industrialization, worldwide overpopulation, artificial contraceptives, prenatal diagnosis, and legalized abortion, the exercise of reproductive responsibility consisted primarily in following the biblical command to "be fruitful and multiply."[1] Assuming that one was legally married, of course, one acted responsibly with regard to reproduction precisely by *having* children. Within some enclaves of the Judeo-Christian tradition, this injunction was no doubt further subjected to a maximizing interpretation: the more children one had, the greater one's degree of responsibility.

Many of us moderns, by contrast, are far more likely to conceive of reproductive responsibility in terms of restraint. In a variety of possible situations, we are inclined to say that someone might act more responsibly precisely by *not* having children, or at least not at this time and in these circumstances. It is important to note here that the invocation of the language of responsibility commits us to a moral point of view with regard to reproductive choice. Instead of viewing the decision whether or not to conceive, bear, and rear a child as primarily or exclusively a matter of individual convenience or unfettered personal choice, many of us are often willing to invoke the moral categories in assessing our own or others' reproductive choices. For example, we might criticize the fifteen-year-old boy for impregnating and then abandoning his girlfriend, while we might praise a family member who, on learning of her carrier status for hemophilia, decides to undergo sterilization rather than risk passing the disease along to future sons.

The advent of artificial contraceptives, especially the birth control pill, gave individual women and couples control over processes that had previously been governed by fate. Prior to the contraceptive revolution a child inopportunely born to parents in their late middle age may have been ruefully accepted as a "gift from God"; but today the birth of such a child might more often be explained as the result of a failure to take proper precautions. Greater control over biological processes has thus engendered a greater sense of personal reproductive responsibility. What can be controlled often should be controlled, especially when failure to do so could entail serious harms or disadvantages to oneself, one's future progeny, or others.

The current arrival of long-term contraceptives represents yet another giant step in the direction of control over nature's unpredictable forces. The insertion of an intrauterine device, the injection of a drug like Depo-Provera, or the surgical implantation of Norplant capsules all provide individual women and couples an unprecedented degree of contraceptive efficiency. In contrast to condoms and diaphragms, which must be used on each occasion of sexual intercourse, and in contrast to the birth control pill, whose effectiveness depends upon daily self-administration, a drug delivery system like Norplant can virtually guarantee a woman or couple a five-year period of extremely efficient contraception, no matter what else the woman or her partners fail to do or refrain from doing. It thus came as no surprise when researchers comparing the effectiveness of Norplant and birth control pills recently found Norplant to be nineteen times more likely than the pill to prevent pregnancy among inner-city, teenage mothers.[2] This is truly artificial contraception on prolonged "automatic pilot."

The good news embodied in such research findings is that individual women and couples desirous of delaying or entirely preventing conception and childbirth now have an extraordinarily powerful tool at their disposal. The more problematical news is that along with this enhanced level of control may well come a heightened sense of moral responsibility to make use of long-term contraceptives. The more we know, and the greater our capacity to predict and eliminate bad consequences, the more we may be expected to avoid those consequences. But clearly the most troubling implication of the availability of long-term contraceptives is that others, and in particular the state, may well be attracted by the extraordinary efficiency of such contraceptives in their own efforts to encourage or, if necessary, to force women to accept such heightened norms of reproductive responsibility. This possibility is by no means merely speculative: we have already seen efforts by judges to require Norplant as a condition of parole for women convicted of child neglect, and efforts by cost-conscious legislators to condition the receipt of welfare benefits upon the acceptance of Norplant by poor women.[3] The great fear, and it is by no means an unreasonable fear, is that the state will put these extraordinarily potent contraceptives in the service not of women's own life plans and reproductive choices, but rather in the service of its own punitive, fiscal, or implicitly discriminatory agendas.

Long-term contraceptives thus promise to be a decidedly mixed blessing. In addition to giving individual women and couples an enhanced ability to control their fertility and hence an expanded range of reproductive liberty, long-term contraceptives also raise in a particularly pressing way disturbing questions about the nature of reproductive responsibility, about the relationship between long-term contraceptives and reproductive responsibility, and about the role of reproductive responsibility in motivating and justifying various social policies, including those that often have greatest impact on poor, vulnerable, and minority women. Although some state-sponsored interventions in the service of reproductive responsibility, such as educational and (some) incentive programs, might well advance the autonomy and well-being of women, other more coercive and punitive approaches may well reflect racist, class-based, or sexist ideologies that threaten to annul women's autonomy in the name of middle-class morality.

In this essay we attempt to come to terms with some of these difficult and disturbing questions. We shall begin with a preliminary analytic account of the nature, grounds, and limits of the concept of reproductive responsibility. We then take up the various uses of this contested concept within three distinct spheres of moral judgment: those of the individual decision maker, the level of moral discourse within a community, and the context of official, public (legislative or judicial) policy. In brief, we shall defend the concept of reproductive responsibility against those who would argue for a notion of unfettered reproductive choice; we commend a suitably hedged conception of reproductive responsibility for purposes of moral assessment and critical dialogue on the individual and social levels; and we close by noting the serious limitations of the concept of reproductive responsibility as a sufficient justification for a variety of problematic social policies.

Reproductive Responsibility: An Analytic Account

In the most general terms, someone acts in a morally irresponsible manner when he or she fails to adequately respond to the needs, interests, or rights of others—that is, the action fails to accord with some standard of good or decent behavior. It is a separate question whether the individual who acts irresponsibly deserves to be blamed for what he or she does, and blame may in fact often be inappropriate for various reasons. An automobile driver who, because he is drunk, injures a pedestrian, has not only acted irresponsibly but is blameworthy as well. Even if, at the time of the accident, he could not exercise sufficient control over his actions to prevent the injury, he either should not have gotten drunk if he was going to drive, or should not have driven if he was going to drink. However, in other cases there may be mitigating or excusing conditions that, while not serving to condone the behavior, make it wrong to condemn, or to condemn as forcefully as we might otherwise have done, the individual for having acted in this way. Thus, it might be argued that we should not blame some women for having children in certain circumstances even if there is a high likelihood that the child will be born with a crippling handicap or a terminal disease. But we might also want to say, and be perfectly justified in saying, that a woman who imposes this risk on her future child is acting irresponsibly, and moreover, that we would be right to blame her for this had the excusing or mitigating factors not been present.[4]

In the next three sections, we set out the main elements of a framework for evaluating procreative choices and acts. We begin with a taxonomy of the objects of irresponsible reproductive conduct—that is, with an examination of the different parties who stand to be harmed or wronged by such conduct. Future children are of course a central concern here, but they are not the only ones who might suffer. Next, we describe a number of critical standards of harm of varying degrees of moral rigor, from "wrongful life" at one extreme to "failure to promote a child's best interests" at the other. The application of these standards, we note, is complicated by the difficulty of measuring likelihood of harm. Finally, we focus on the individuals themselves whose procreative acts violate these standards and on the factors that might render blame, or full blame, inappropriate. In the section on "Multiculturalism and Reproductive Responsibility," we discuss the various ways in which the application of our analytic framework is affected by the existence of cultural differences.

The Objects of Irresponsible Reproduction

First, one can act irresponsibly by shirking one's parental duties and unfairly shifting the burden of child rearing to others. The teenage boy who fathers a child only to abandon both child and mother acts irresponsibly in this way. So too does the young woman who, consumed by her drug habit, has a child knowing full well that her own aging mother will have to assume the role of primary caretaker, even though she is unprepared or unwilling to do so. In the latter case, it makes sense to say that the young woman's reproductive behavior is irresponsible, for even though the child will have someone to take care of it and will not be abandoned, raising a child at this time in her mother's life constitutes an unwelcome intrusion and burden. The young woman, we might say, is acting irresponsibly toward or with regard to her own mother.

Second, one might plausibly claim that a young person can act irresponsibly with regard to herself or himself by having a child if, by doing so, she or he thereby forecloses important opportunities for personal development. Though some philosophers find difficulty with the notion of having duties to oneself, we believe that individuals are responsible to themselves for what they make of their lives and that they may be showing a sort of disrespect for themselves if, especially during their formative years, they act in ways that severely restrict their life prospects. Consider, for example, the teenage girl who has barely begun high school, for whom having and raising a child would mean the interruption of her education, the derailing of her life plans, and the forgoing of opportunities to develop her full potential. Whatever we might say about the future child's quality of life, she owes it to herself not to have a child at this time.

Third, a person or couple contemplating having an additional child might act irresponsibly toward their already existing children if their welfare would be severely diminished by the added burdens of child rearing. Consider a young couple on the fringe of poverty who are just barely able to meet the physical and emotional needs of their five children. If they were to have yet another child, it would be virtually impossible for them properly to feed, clothe, house, or nurture their other existing children. Yet the claims of the new child do not take precedence over the claims of those for whom they are already responsible, and it would be irresponsible of the parents to endanger the other children in this way.

Fourth, many believe that one of the victims of irresponsible reproduction is society itself. When parents are incapable of adequately rearing their children on their own, society must step in to protect the welfare of children, and this, it is alleged, places a burden on the other members of society that they should not have had to bear. However, this view may be contested. It fails to address the reality that many of these parents are not able to do a decent job raising their children because society has in various ways failed to give them the resources and assistance they need to be able to do so.

Finally, charges of reproductive irresponsibility are based on concerns about the welfare of the children one is bringing into the world. If the child's existence falls below some threshold of acceptable well-being, then it would have been better had the child not been born at all, and in some cases one can be blamed for reproducing if one knows this is likely to happen. The critical question, of course, is how to define this threshold.

There are, to sum up, multiple parties who might be wronged or harmed by irresponsible reproduction: future and existing children, individuals who become primary caretakers by default, the procreators themselves, and possibly society at large. But while there may be general agreement that harm or wrong to the future child can ground a charge of irresponsible reproduction, there is considerably less agreement on what the standard of harm or wrong should be here. This is the problem to which we now turn.

Critical Standards of Harm to Future Children

Sometimes it is wrong to reproduce because there is a risk either that the child will be born in a condition harmful to it or that the child, once born, will later be harmed. Judgments of this sort depend on two kinds of standards, one that identifies the nature of the harm and the other that sets a threshhold for acceptable risk. In other words, the wrongfulness of reproduction is a function not of potential harm alone, but of the particular mix of harm and risk in a given case. Several combinations of harm and risk are possible—small or significant risk and moderate or grave harm—and it is plausible to suppose that different combinations will have different implications for the wrongfulness of reproducing under these conditions. We will say something about assessment of risk after we complete our classification of standards of harm.

For some theorists, the notion of *wrongful life* marks the dividing line between responsible and irresponsible reproductive behavior toward future children.[5] Cases of so-called wrongful life are those rare instances in which a child's life prospects are so bleak or compromised as to render his or her life not worth living. In these cases, any rational observer would judge that it would have been better that a child had never existed than to suffer in such a diminished state. A child born in such a state is perhaps not, strictly speaking, "harmed" by being born, since he is not put in a worse condition thereby than he would otherwise be in, for otherwise he would not have been at all. Nevertheless, proponents of the wrongful life view claim that such a child is "wronged" by the parents' decision to procreate.

In order to apply the wrongful life standard, we have to be able to identify those handicaps which are so severe that, in the words of Joel Feinberg, "they doom a child's most basic future interests to defeat."[6] A child who is doomed to spend his life in a persistent vegetative state, or in severe and intractable pain, would seem to have been wronged by being born. But beyond this, consensus unravels. Even with a disease like Tay-Sachs, for example, there are people who find the affliction to be unfortunate in the extreme but not an injustice visited upon the child by his or her parents. What seems clear is that while there may be certain conditions that all rational, caring observers would judge make "life worth living" impossible, their number is exceedingly small. And this is important for the following reason: most of the conditions that prompt people to worry about reproductive responsibility would not be covered by a wrongful life standard, such as being born in abject poverty or to a drug-addicted mother.

Were wrongful life the *only* legitimate criterion of irresponsible reproductive behavior toward future children, then hardly any procreative acts could be deemed truly irresponsible. No matter how badly off any particular child happened to be, no matter how sick or debilitated or socially isolated, no matter how short her anticipated life span, her parents would do nothing wrong by bringing her into existence as long as the child's life could be thought minimally worth living.[7] And this will lead many to conclude that wrongful life cannot be the only way to fix the threshold of acceptable well-being for future children.

To accommodate such cases, we need to supplement the wrongful life standard with what we call the *grievous burdens* standard—i.e., the view that reproductive choices and acts can be irresponsible when the resulting child is likely to lead a life of extremely poor quality or short duration, or both, but that is not necessarily wrongful. Imagine a world in which a prenatal test were available to detect the presence of a mysterious new disease in a fetus with 100 percent accuracy, yet in which no effective treatments had been developed to treat those infants affected by the disease. Suppose further that in this imaginary scenario all affected children would suffer from recurring infections and other medical problems and would die of the disease before they reached the age of seven. Many of these children, however, could enjoy life with their families and friends, both at home and at school, in between bouts of serious illness in the hospital. At the end of their brief lives, most of these children ruefully admit that despite their affliction, they do not wish they had never been born. Nevertheless, considering the suffering these children would undergo, reproducing in the face of predictable and extremely grievous burdens like these seems only marginally less troubling than reproducing in the face of wrongful life.

Reproduction can be irresponsible not only because the child will be born with physical and psychological handicaps, but also because the child, even if born healthy, will receive inadequate care. Though parents in our society are to a large extent free to raise their children as they deem best, children are not their parents' property: they have welfare rights, both positive and negative, that place moral constraints on the exercise of parental authority. What these positive rights consist of and what they require of parents in the way of conditions for their satisfaction are matters about which there is some dispute, but there is widespread agreement on certain minimum requirements of decent parenting. Parents who engage in abusive or neglectful behavior, in the sense of gross physical injury and severe deprivation, are deemed unfit. So too are those parents who subject their children to severe emotional abuse and neglect—who, for example, are never emotionally available to them or constantly belittle their achievements and strivings. (Since it is extremely difficult to predict when a child is emotionally endangered or to recognize instances of emotional harm, this is a shaky foundation upon which to justify coercive state intervention. But this is a separate issue to which we shall return in the section on "Employing Norms of Reproductive Responsibility.")

Abuse and neglect are here defined in terms of actual or likely harmful consequences for the child—not parental intentions—and it is only parental behavior that is extremely detrimental to the physical or psychological health or well-being of the child that is being labeled abusive or neglectful. Definitions of abuse and neglect are possible that do not view harmful consequences for the child as the critical factor, and these may be preferable for certain purposes. But by limiting ourselves to what we take to be the least controversial way of understanding these notions, we can formulate a standard of reproductive responsibility that has broad public appeal. We call this the *abuse/neglect standard*: reproductive behavior is criticizable when the child who is born will subsequently be physically or emotionally abused or neglected. Moreover, when individuals can reasonably be expected to foresee that having a child in certain circumstances will lead to its abuse or neglect, then—absent excusing conditions—they can be blamed for reproducing. If they engage in sexual relations and cannot countenance abortion, or regard it as morally problematic, then for the sake of the child, they ought to take steps to prevent pregnancy.

Parents who abuse or neglect their children do not just fail to give them a good upbringing. Rather, they fail to give them a minimally acceptable one. Children have certain needs that must be met at least to some extent, and in any community the terms "abusive" and "neglectful" are reserved for the most egregious violations of standards of parenting. However, even if there is widespread agreement on some minimum requirements of parenting, in a pluralistic, culturally diverse society there may be substantial disagreement on others. For example, the Amish community and many in so-called mainstream society disagree on what is appropriate education for children. The sort of education that the Amish maintain is necessary to preserve their traditional way of life others regard as a deprivation of the rights of the children. What is being claimed here is not that Amish parents are physically or emotionally abusing or neglecting their children, but rather that they are *failing to meet their minimum needs*.

The general form of the abuse/neglect standard is this: if it is wrong for parents to treat (or raise) their child in a certain way, then it is wrong for them to have a child when they will treat (or raise) it in this way. Additional standards can be formulated that have the same form, but are more morally rigorous. Thus, suppose parents act irresponsibly if their behavior is not in the *best interests* of their children—that is, if it fails to optimize their child's potential for a good or fulfilling life. Then it follows from the general standard for reproductive irresponsibility that parents who will fail to promote their child's best interests do wrong to have the child. However, it seems to us unreasonable to speak of reproductive irresponsibility in these cases, since a standard requiring parents to optimize their child's potential imposes extraordinary burdens on parents who have their own lives to lead and perhaps other responsibilities as well. What's more, attributions of irresponsibility based on the best interests standard are particularly susceptible to being influenced by the personal values and biases of those doing the judging.

In summary, the wrongful life standard and the best interests standard are at opposite extremes on a continuum of norms of reproductive irresponsibility. Very few (too few) instances of reproductive behavior would be judged irresponsible if only the former standard were used, and many more instances (too many, we think) would be judged irresponsible if the latter test were used. The wrongful life, grievous burdens, and abuse/neglect standards seem to us to specify conditions under which a charge of wrongful reproduction is justified. The minimum needs standard, however, is more problematic, since even if there is general agreement on what a child needs, it may be more difficult to determine what constitutes a mimimum level of satisfaction of these needs. And finally we believe that the best interest standard is objectionable because it imposes unreasonably demanding obligations on parents and disregards competing interests or rights, such as those of parents themselves or of siblings.

Risk

Charges of reproductive irresponsibility, we said earlier, must be grounded not only in some notion of what constitutes harm, but also in an assessment of the *risk* of harm that is imposed by, or that follows upon, the act of procreation. We have so far bracketed this problem in order to simplify the exposition, but it must be emphasized that our willingness to criticize reproductive behavior often turns on this very issue. For example, the probability of an HIV-positive woman transmitting HIV to her child is approximately 8% if the woman takes AZT during pregnancy and the child receives it during the first several months of life; the risk of transmitting a genetic disease like Tay-Sachs, if both parents are carriers, is 25%. Are the risks of imposing the grievous burdens of these diseases on offspring morally unacceptable? And how likely must it be that parents will abuse or neglect their child before we say that the risk is too high and that those who reproduce under these circumstances are acting irresponsibly? The likelihood that parents will be abusive or neglectful depends on numerous psychological, familial, and social factors, and this further complicates the task of assessing reproductive responsibility.

As mentioned earlier, there are two separate evaluations in any judgment about a given risk: one measures the gravity of the worst possible outcome, the other perceives whether a given probability is great or small. For devastating diseases like AIDS and Tay-Sachs, and for gross physical abuse and severe deprivation, the first part of the judgment should be unproblematic. In these cases, the pain and suffering the child endures substantially impair his opportunity for a good life. As for the second part of the judgment, people may regard the same probability of an uncontestedly bad outcome quite differently. Some might believe that, say, an 8% probability of transmitting HIV is not too great; others might believe that under these circumstances, they should either remain childless or seek nonstandard ways of creating a family.

If an individual's or a couple's parental desires can equally well be satisfied by nonstandard ways of creating a family—e.g., by adoption or some forms of assisted reproduction—as by childbearing that poses a risk of serious disability, then plainly they are criticizable if they reproduce. But this is probably seldom the case, and there will often be individuals for whom having their own child is so important that a statistically significant probability of transmitting a serious handicap to their offspring is no deterent to reproduction. We do not believe that a principled argument can be given for fixing the threshold of tolerable risk for responsible childbearing at 10%, 25%, or 50%. These specific cutoffs lack an underlying theoretical rationale and are thus essentially arbitrary. However, the following more modest position seems unexceptionable: as the likelihood of harm (including but not limited to the harm of inherited handicaps) to the offspring becomes more certain, the greater becomes the burden of showing that one is not acting irresponsibly by reproducing.

Assigning Blame

Wrongdoing is one of the components of reproductive irresponsibility, and individuals do wrong to reproduce if they cause a child to exist who is likely to be harmed (as determined by one of the above standards) either by the act of procreation itself or by further parental behavior. But faulting the *act* is one thing and faulting the *agent* for acting in a certain way is quite another, and various factors can absolve a person of blame, or blunt the force of blame, even when the conduct he or she engages in is itself objectionable. We now discuss some of these, dividing them into the following categories:

circumstances of conception and birth, burdens of foregoing childbearing, and psychological handicaps.

Circumstances of conception and birth

We mention under this heading three examples: contraceptive failure, lack of resources, and personal pressures. First, consider a couple who believe correctly that it would be wrong of them to reproduce—either at this time or at all—and who use contraceptives in a responsible manner. Despite these precautions, however, a fetus is conceived, and since they have strong religious or moral objections to abortion, they have the child. If the initial decision not to have a child was based only on beliefs about the sort of upbringing they would give it, they have the option of trying to find another caretaker for their offspring. But suppose instead that it was based on legitimate worries about having a severely handicapped child, and that as it turns out, this is the child they have. Should the couple be blamed for reproducing? On the one hand, no one compelled them to have the child: it was their voluntary choice. Yet on the other, they did take precautions to avoid pregnancy, and these having failed, they were not exactly free to discard their convictions about abortion. Given these convictions, there is a sense in which they could do no other than to go ahead and have the child. It seems plausible to say that while such parents may not be totally blameless—they did, after all, assume a serious risk—they are far less to blame than parents who were irresponsible about the use of contraceptives or who did not have strong objections to abortion.

A second factor that may mitigate blame for having a child, or perhaps absolve parents of blame, has to do with the parents' lack of access to resources and services that can help ameliorate the conditions that contribute to abuse and neglect of children. These conditions include poverty, unemployment, and lack of education. Many parents who abuse or neglect their children could be significantly helped by such aids as more money, better housing, employment counseling or training, family planning counseling, and child care services of various sorts. But large numbers of individuals may lack access to these resources because of social and economic policies and practices that are both unwise and unjust. If women have children in spite of the threat of serious harm or their own inability to care for them, and if they do this in large measure because of the unavailability of necessary information and services, then it makes much more sense to blame society rather than these women for failures of reproductive responsibility. Even members of the middle class who are justifiably impatient with the currently fashionable celebration of victimhood can and should recognize that such women are more justly viewed as victims of social neglect than as intentional wrongdoers.

Third, individuals might be subjected to personal pressures of various sorts to have a child—from relatives, lovers, and others—and this too can affect how harshly we ought to judge those who reproduce irresponsibly, or whether we ought to judge them at all. One thinks here of women in various African countries who are placed under enormous social and familial pressures to have children, or of women in various minority communities in the United States who are subjected to similar, if perhaps somewhat less intense, societal expectations.

Burdens of foregoing childbirth

People want to have children for all sorts of reasons: to have someone to love and be loved by, to give their lives a sense of purpose, to elevate their status within the community, to extend the genetic line, to be surrounded by replicas of themselves, and so on. In traditional cultures, moreover, couples often have children primarily to provide labor for the family farm. Some of these desires, since they are really desires to parent rather than to bear a child, can be satisfied by nonstandard ways of creating a family, and if normal procreation risked harm to the offspring, we would hope that such alternative methods were available to individuals. (Indeed, perhaps society ought to do more than hope and work to make such methods available through provision of subsidies for adoption and the like.) But in some cases, individuals might not have access to nonstandard ways of satisfying their desires pertaining to family life, or they might have strong desires that cannot be met by these methods. Indeed, a woman might truly believe that her sense of identity and worth derive exclusively from her ability to bear children. (We return to this point in the section on "Multiculturalism and Reproductive Responsibility.") For these individuals, there is no meaningful or genuine alternative to normal procreation if they want to become parents, and forgoing this might constitute a serious hardship for them. It might still be the case, of course, that the reproductively responsible thing to do under the circumstances is not to reproduce. But the sort of hardship and sacrifice they would have to endure if they refrained from procreating might be such as to render blame, or at least full blame, inappropriate.

Psychological handicaps

If individuals cannot reasonably be expected to know that, should they decide to reproduce, the resulting child may have a serious handicap or will be at risk of harm, then a necessary condition of assigning blame is not met. Severely mentally retarded individuals who reproduce fall in this category, as do those who, through no fault of their own, are grossly ignorant of the risks to which they subject their future child. In other cases, blame is at least mitigated because the individuals involved, though biologically mature, are so psychologically immature that they cannot appreciate the risks they pose by reproducing or foresee what they are letting themselves in for by having a child. Many adolescents, for example, are still children themselves, psychologically incapable of appreciating the long-term consequences of their procreative choices. And finally, it is inappropriate to hold individuals fully morally responsible for their reproductive acts if their ability to exercise control over their behavior is substantially impaired by drug addiction or mental illness.

Multiculturalism and Reproductive Responsibility

The task of applying norms of responsible reproduction in the context of a pluralistic social order like ours is complicated by the fact that such a society tolerates—even encourages—diverse ways of life among its members. (A "way of life," as we are using the term, is shared by the members of a group and consists of a particular configuration of moral, religious, philosophical, and/ or cultural values and beliefs.) One of the implications of this attitude to diversity is that individuals have the right, within broad limits, to make decisions affecting the welfare of their children that reflect and reinforce the particular system of basic beliefs and values that guides the parents' own lives. Moreover, respect for diversity in ways of life demands that parents not be labeled irresponsible merely because their decisions are guided by a belief system that other groups in society do not share. Indeed, if those applying our basic framework pretend that their own perspective on reproductive responsibility somehow represents a universal, unbiased, "view from nowhere,"[8] it is highly likely that their conclusions will be both ideologically tainted and profoundly disrespectful of the agents being judged. Although we do not rule out the possibility that truly universal moral norms might be exist, a sober assessment of the historical record indicates that most explicit pretentions to universality usually function implicitly as smokescreens for the very particular agenda of a certain race, class, or sex.

The application of our analytic framework to the gamut of reproductive choices and behavior thus requires a careful consideration of relevant cultural differences. Indeed, each of the three major elements of our framework— i.e., the nature and magnitude of potential harms, their likelihood of occurring, and the components of blame—is fair game for a searching multicultural critique and reinterpretation.[9] Beginning with the nature and magnitude of the threatened harm, one could argue that those standing within a culture of poverty, deprivation, and racial discrimination might see certain kinds of harms—such as being born HIV positive or without a father—as somehow less ominous than the inhabitants of white, middle-class culture would view them. Many HIV-positive women, for example, tend to place the fate of their future children in the hands of God. Should their child turn out to be infected, many such women might well see this as just one more misfortune heaped upon their life—as a misfortune willed, or at least permitted, by a loving God and not, therefore, as something to be avoided at all costs.

By the same token, one's attitude toward the likelihood of risk and the burdens of forgoing parenthood are profoundly influenced by culture and class. Those whose lives are relatively comfortable and risk free often tend to see the reproductive glass as being half empty, while those whose daily surroundings are more threatening may well tend to see it as half full. Thus, women living with the daily risks of drug addiction, partner abuse, or homelessness might be more likely to see the 25% risk of passing HIV or a genetic anomaly on to their children as a 75% chance of having a much-loved normal baby.

And in spite of the fact that many people now tend to view reproductive responsibility in terms of restraint rather than productivity, many women are still profoundly influenced by the cultural belief, recently labelled by one observer as the philosophy of "maternalism," that having children is always and everywhere a good thing, and that our sole responsibility with regard to reproduction is simply to have children and take care of them as well as one is able.[10] Women influenced by this widespread cultural belief, women whose very identities are fused with the prospect of giving birth and mothering, will find it particularly burdensome to forgo having children. Such women can be found not merely in various inner-city or rural subcultural pockets, but also in the waiting rooms of in vitro fertilization clinics exclusively serving a middle- and upper-class clientele in mainstream America.

Having acknowledged the existence and importance of such cultural factors, we must now ask exactly what role they should play in our moral assessments. One response, which we shall call "hard-core multiculturalism," holds that cultural differences undercut the very possibility of assigning moral praise and blame to people and behaviors occupying a different cultural space than one's own. At bottom a contemporary variant of moral and cultural relativism, this view contends that all moral values are the product of particular cultures, that they have validity only within their natal settings, and that cross-cultural moral judgments are therefore inappropriate and disrespectful of the people being judged. In the context of recent debates over the appropriateness of HIV-infected women having children, for example, some hard-core multiculturalists have claimed that white, middle-class professionals simply have no business judging and trying to influence the reproductive choices of poor women of color.[11]

Although we acknowledge the existence and importance of cultural and class differences, we find hard-core multiculturalism to be a deeply problematic and ultimately untenable moral response. When confronted by such differences, this brand of multiculturalism would not only rule out "us" criticizing "them," no matter how unethical or inhuman we think their behavior to be, but it would also reassure us that we need not take seriously any criticism levelled at us by them. Both of these postures, we would argue, unnecessarily constrict the range of fruitful moral discourse.

This is so for either of two reasons. First, we might sincerely believe that the practices of another culture or subculture violate universal human rights. For example, some critics of female genital mutilation in various Muslim countries hold that this practice violates the rights of the affected young girls and women to health and sexual satisfaction.[12] Conversely, both the foreign and Northern critics of slavery in the pre–Civil war American South no doubt often argued that this practice violated fundamental rights.[13] Contrary to both of these powerful moral appeals, hard-core multiculturalism would preclude moral criticism on either front. It would reassure the mutilators and exploiters of both women and slaves that they need not listen to this disturbing moral noise coming from the outside.

Second, even granting the existence of some important cultural differences among the various groups composing our society, it is a serious mistake to assume that we all exist in rigidly defined cultural compartments, each one hermetically sealed off from all the others. The fact is that in a pluralistic and cosmopolitan society like ours—a society, we might add, in which network television is, for better or worse, the national educator—most of us tend to inhabit a wide variety of intersecting roles and cultures, and we often share values that cut across our differences, even on matters as fundamental as reproduction. Although it would often be a mistake to assume convergence around mainstream values, it would also be a mistake to assume that the many differences separating, say, poor women of color from middle-class professionals necessarily entail serious differences about the meaning and importance of childbearing and child rearing. As Anita Allen observes in a thoughtful article on HIV and reproduction,[14] poor women of color not only share middle-class white women's embrace of "maternalism," but they also on occasion give voice to concerns that we might expect from white professionals. Allen cites some poor, black women as saying, for example, that it is a "sin" to bring an HIV-infected baby into the world, that one "must think of their little lives . . . when they don't have anything," and that HIV-infected women have to ask themselves if they will "be there" for their child.

There is a sense, then, in which—all our differences notwithstanding—we all inhabit large expanses of the same cultural space within which we can talk with each other and even on occasion criticize each other. But hardcore multiculturalism fails us even in the presence of serious differences and disagreements between cultures and within the subcultures of a single political state. Even if one denies the existence of universal human rights, fruitful dialogue and moral judgment are still often possible across cultural boundaries. This kind of dialogue, however, requires a great deal of hard work. Instead of simply imposing some universal moral law on the occupants of some other culture or subculture, this option requires us to enter the world of the "other," to "walk in her shoes," to see the world as she sees it. It requires a tremendous effort at translation of our moral vocabulary and values into theirs, and of theirs into ours. In the words of the German philosopher Hans Georg Gadamer, it requires a "fusion of horizons," neither of which is necessarily privileged.[15]

Once we have achieved an adequate understanding of the other culture, once this fusion of intellectual and moral horizons has been accomplished, criticism might still be possible, but it will have to rest on a set of values that have been enriched or even transformed by the encounter with the other.[16] Thus, having immersed ourselves in the lives and culture of others, "we" might point out to "them" that a particularly repulsive practice of theirs is not necessarily dictated by their holy scriptures and yet causes great physical suffering, while "they" might teach "us" that some of our most firmly entrenched attitudes and beliefs—for example, our idolatry of the handgun—are equally dehumanizing and destructive.[17] In addition, once we have made a serious effort to understand another culture on its own terms, we may find that abundant resources already exist in that culture for criticizing behavior that violates our own norms of right and wrong. Instead of attempting to carry out a cross-cultural critique with the aid of standards that might seem completely foreign to our interlocutors, we may come to know enough about a culture to criticize some of its practices in terms that will be entirely familiar to its members. In such situations the motivation to criticize would naturally come from our own cultural understandings, but the linguistic, conceptual, and normative medium of our criticism would be provided by the alternative culture. The general form of such criticism is to show that the challenged conduct or practice actually violates norms to which a people are already committed.[18] The charge, in effect, is one of inconsistency or even hypocrisy.

In sum, we do not need universal moral norms in order to teach and learn from each other. Indeed, the hasty and insensitive invocation of such norms will often preclude the possibility of precisely this kind of salutary teaching and learning. Instead, we need to be open and attentive to ways in which our particular values might, once suitably translated, find resonances and points of contact in the other culture.

Notwithstanding its failure to provide an adequate moral standpoint, our examination of hard-core multiculturalism teaches valuable lessons about the positive contributions of a more modest critical multiculturalism. The first of these is that once we have taken the full array of cultural differences into account, individual blame may not be the most appropriate or helpful moral response to difference.[19] If the reproductive behavior of individuals is shaped by widely and intensely held cultural beliefs, it is both inappropriate and counterproductive to begin a dialogue by heaping blame on them. Even if "we" are convinced that "they" are not being sufficiently responsive to the needs of others, including their own future progeny, we must acknowledge that they may well be acting in good conscience. One can, of course, act out of good conscience and still be wrong, but being wrong is not the same as being blameworthy.

The second lesson, really a corollary of the first, is that an awareness of cultural difference should make us much less quick to judge. Once we realize that the vast majority of our most deeply entrenched moral views reflect thickly interpreted "local" understandings based upon our own way of life,[20] we then see clearly that our first instinct should not be to judge or cast moral blame, but rather to attempt to understand the problematic belief or behavior in the context of its own localized meanings. Once we have done that, once our moral horizons have expanded and fused with those of the other, we may still want to engage in moral judgment. But reserving the right to judge, once one has truly understood, is not the same as being judgmental.[21]

A third implication of multiculturalism, closely related to the last, concerns our theory of the virtues required for the good life. Once we see that our notion of the good life requires that it be lived alongside of others within pluralistic, multicultural, and increasingly cosmopolitan societies, we are ready to acknowledge an expanded role for the virtues of humility and empathy. While empathy has long occupied an honored place in the pantheon of moral virtues, especially within its utilitarian wing, humility has often been relegated to the pantheon's storeroom, a throwback to the bygone days of a breast-beating, hair-shirted Christianity.[22] But within the context of contemporary multicultural societies, humility becomes a pivotal moral virtue, conditioning our all-important initial responses to morally troubling differences.

The final lesson of multiculturalism for our theory of reproductive responsibility, one not sufficiently appreciated in the multicultural literature, stems from the *failure* of its hard-core variant: notwithstanding the particular and localized nature of most of our moral concepts and vocabulary, communication and critique across cultures is still possible.[23] Contrary to the claim of hard-core multiculturalists that moral criticism across cultural or subcultural boundaries is inappropriate and disrespectful, we would argue that nothing could be more disrespectful to other people as rational agents than precisely this hands-off attitude. For when we say that people of other cultures should not be engaged, praised, or criticized, we imply that they are, in a sense, *merely* the products of their environment and that they lack the critical ability to step back from their own history and traditions to ask about their merit and possible faults. We believe that it shows much more concern and respect for the moral agency and cultural traditions of others to take them seriously enough to learn their moral language, to participate—to the extent possible—in their way of seeing things, and to engage them in an ever-widening dialogue into the nature of the good and the right.

Employing Norms of Reproductive Responsibility

The analytic discussion of reproductive responsibility starts from the assumption that the reproductive choices of individuals are properly the object of moral evaluation and, potentially, moral criticism. If this were not the case, and if reproductive decisions were assimilable to decisions based on personal preference or taste, then the search for specific moral standards or mitigating factors would be a waste of time. But the claim that reproductive choices are of the sort that makes moral scrutiny appropriate is deeply troubling to many people, and this, we believe, is due in large measure to the connection they make between moral criticism and coercive legal intervention. Charges of reproductive irresponsibility are seen, often with good reason, as paving the way for some form of state interference with reproductive freedom. But the connection here is practical, not conceptual, and the objection to certain kinds of state action carries no implication at all about the possibility and validity of passing moral judgment on people's reproductive choices. Judging that it would be morally irresponsible of this person or couple to have a child is one thing, advocating state coercion to prevent childbearing is quite another. The latter is only one of a number of possible uses of the notion of reproductive responsibility, some of which we will now discuss.

Personal Decision Making

To begin with, the notion of reproductive responsibility also figures in the personal decision making of individual women and men. Even those who maintain that reproductive choices are not the moral business of anyone other than the individuals involved might judge for themselves that it would be an irresponsible act on their part to have a child at a certain time in their lives because of what this will mean in terms of their own life prospects, the well-being of their child, or the required sacrifices on the part of other caretakers. In order more clearly to grasp this point, imagine the internal monologue of a teenager endowed with a heightened moral sensitivity as she confronts an array of reproductive choices. She reasons that at the age of fifteen she is not ready to be a parent. She needs to do her own growing up before she can be a good mother to her children. To have children now, she thinks, would in a sense be unfair to them; they deserve a better start in life. And so does she: this young woman would much rather finish school and get a job or go to college than start having babies in her mid-teens. Since she admits to herself that she is either unwilling or unable to abstain entirely from sexual intercourse with her boyfriends, she must have recourse to some kind of contraceptive drug or device. Which to choose? Assuming that in her case the likely adverse health effects of the pill and Norplant are more or less equivalent—of course, a very big "if"—and that Norplant is roughly nineteen times more effective than the pill,[24] our teen might well conclude that the most morally responsible course of action open to her is to opt for Norplant. Indeed, given her candid self-assessment as a typical teenager likely to go off the pill after a year and face the high likelihood of an unwanted pregnancy, she may well come to see opting for the pill as a relatively irresponsible act.

To be sure, the efficiency of such drugs could never by itself settle the issue of the most responsible method of contraception for her to use. Should such contraceptives pose significant health, financial, or other risks to this young woman, she would certainly have to consider such factors in her own personal decision-making calculus. If the risks were at all palpable and significant, no one could reasonably claim that her decision not to expose herself to them would be irresponsible, even if in doing so she were to forgo some measure of additional contraceptive security.

Communal Standards of Conduct

But reproductive responsibility is not, after all, exclusively a private concern, and the notion has a use that extends beyond the province of private decision making. It is also used by society or a community to express its shared sense of what is morally correct or praiseworthy in reproductive matters, and there is nothing in principle objectionable about this. In spite of the fact that in our society reproductive decisions are often portrayed as existing exclusively within the purview of individual judgment and discretion—as private matters on which others have no business passing moral judgment—this is a false and impoverished picture. There are, as we noted earlier, victims of reproductive irresponsibility, including other potential care-takers, existing children, and the future children themselves. This moves reproduction out of the private domain and into the sphere of what John Stuart Mill referred to as "other regarding behavior"—that is, conduct that can affect the morally significant interests of others in profoundly detrimental ways.

Though the content of norms of responsible procreative behavior may vary considerably from one community to another, such norms do in fact exist in most communities of which we are aware. The community might be the dominant group within a particular society or only a small and relatively powerless minority, but the community to which one belongs sets standards for one's conduct. Should a woman or a couple impose a risk of disease or genetic anomaly upon their offspring that exceeds the bounds of reasonable discretion within their moral community, whatever those bounds might be, they are subject to moral blame on the part of other members of that community. Similar things are said on a regular basis within moral communities regarding other varieties of reproductive irresponsibility. Thus, a drug-addicted woman who imposes child-rearing responsibilities on her aging mother might, within certain communities, be harshly judged as being thoughtless, selfish, and irresponsible, as might parents who have an extra child in the face of evidence of their inability to properly care for their already existing children. At the same time, women or couples are also praised for their exercise of reproductive responsibility in refraining from having children in appropriate circumstances. To be sure, reproductive decisions have a private and intensely personal aspect. But the notion of reproductive responsibility reaches beyond the private domain and inevitably and properly figures in the social morality of a community.

This is not to suggest that a particular community must be so homogeneous that there will never be disagreements within it about how to specify its norms or about which practices best promote the community's sense of reproductive responsibility. It is even possible that a small but powerful minority within a community will attempt to project its own narrow but passionately felt sense of morality and responsibility on the rest of the commu-nity, falsely identifying its own morality with that of the larger, more heteroge-nous group. This *may* be an accurate account of what happened in Baltimore when local ministers intervened to prevent young women and their parents from requesting the availability of Norplant in the public school system.

Moreover, a community's sense of what counts as responsible reproductive behavior may be ethically flawed. A particular community, for example, might obstinately cling to a practice that formerly tended to enrich the lives of its members, but which has been rendered obsolete or even harmful by changed external circumstances. Any full-blown response to Anita Allen's thesis that a widespread "philosophy of maternalism" not only absolves all HIV-infected women of moral blame, but actually puts their conduct out of reach of further moral assessment,[25] would have to begin here. Although this is not the place to pursue this point, we would argue that such a "maternalist" understanding ignores crucial contextual features of reproductive responsibility, such as the prospect of serious harm to others and to future children, the ability to foresee and prevent such harms through reproductive restraint and the diagnostic and treatment capabilities of contemporary medicine, and the availability of freely chosen contraception and abortion.

Finally, as noted above, the values of the community might be questioned on more universalistic grounds of individual autonomy, human rights, or social justice. The parents of young women and girls in many Muslim countries of Africa and the Middle East, for example, are taught that subjecting their daughters to genital mutilation is the height of sexual responsibility. For this and all the above reasons, one should be careful not to read too much into our claim that the language of reproductive responsibility is an important part of communal moral discourse. Although they shape all particular conceptions of reproductive responsibility, the current values of any given community always remain open to critical scrutiny.

Public Policy

A third use of the notion of reproductive responsibility is to motivate some form of state intervention into the reproductive decisions of individuals. Such intervention may be either noncoercive, as in various educational or incentive programs, or coercive, as in the form of threats to condition continuing receipt of welfare benefits on the use of a long-term contraceptive. Although noncoercive modalities of state intervention pose fewer moral problems than frankly coercive programs, both merit the most careful scrutiny.

Although the term "coercion" remains a difficult and contested moral concept,[26] we consider both a broad range of educational efforts and various incentive programs to be noncoercive and probably the best candidates for justifiable state intervention on grounds of reproductive responsibility. We see no problem, for example, with educational messages aimed at all teenagers to stay in school, refrain from childbearing, and develop their own skills and abilities until such time as they can be good parents—or at least better parents than they would have been at the age of fifteen or sixteen. Operating as they do through appeals to rationality, self-interest, and the interest of their future children, and enjoying as they do the widest possible consensus across the societal spectrum, such educational messages appear to be strongly justified.[27]

Naturally, coercive interventions pose even greater problems and warrant even closer scrutiny. First, different communities within the larger society may espouse different norms of reproductive responsibility or different interpretations of common norms, and there may not be sufficient social consensus around a norm or its interpretation to justify its authoritative enforcement by coercive legal measures. For example, even if different moral communities espoused a "failure to meet minimum needs" standard of reproductive responsibility, it would be naive to suppose that in a society in which diversity is respected there would be total agreement on what constitutes a minimal level of satisfaction of children's needs.

Second, the justification of coercive state intervention in reproduction depends on more than showing that an individual's or couple's reproductive decisions run afoul of some standard of reproductive responsibility, even supposing that the standard in question is widely accepted in society and clearly applies to the case at hand. If, for example, it can reasonably be predicted that having a child in certain circumstances will likely lead to its abuse or neglect, and the state is justified in coercively intervening in the parent-child relationship to protect a child from abuse or neglect, it may be thought that the state is also justified in coercively intervening before birth to prevent future abuse and neglect. It must be recalled, however, that intervening in the prenatal period is far more ethically and legally complicated in view of the parents' countervailing rights of reproductive liberty—rights which weigh heavily before but not after birth.

Forcing potential child abusers to use long-acting contraceptives would prevent the abuse of any future children, but it would do so by precluding the man or woman from having children. This is an extreme response to the problem of child abuse, because there are other less intrusive measures that could be taken to prevent such harm, such as therapy, instruction in parenting skills, heightened supervision, and so on. (In addition, forced contraception does not address the root causes of most child abuse and cannot be justified as therapeutic for the individuals who have committed or are likely to commit child abuse.) In general, then, even if we as a society agree that it would be wrong for persons to have children they are likely to abuse, this does not entail that state coercive intervention to prevent reproduction is morally justified.

A third reason to be wary of state intervention to enforce reproductive responsibility has to do with the fact that this notion encompasses more than a concern for the interests of future children. Reproduction might be judged irresponsible, we have argued, because of the damage it will do to the lives of the procreators, because of the extreme hardship it will cause for already existing children, or because of the unfair demands it will place on other caretakers within the family circle. But clearly the state is in no position to determine what any potential parent owes herself or himself, what is the breaking point for a family in terms of additional children, and who within a family ought to be shielded from additional caretaking duties. Were the state given the right to investigate these matters and then coercively intervene in reproductive decisions on one of these grounds, the result would surely be a massive and utterly intolerable intrusion into the sphere of family autonomy and privacy.

Conclusion

A proper concern for reproductive responsibility can thus motivate a broad range of discussions and interventions bearing on the reproductive choices of individuals. The ultimate wisdom or justifiability of any such intervention, however, will depend on a complex web of other judgments bearing on typical social policy concerns, such as efficiency, political feasibility, necessity (i.e., can the same result be achieved in other, less intrusive ways?), fairness, and the policy's impact on moral or human rights. In our judgment, very few of the proposed policy uses of long-term contraceptives pass these latter tests.

But even if notions of reproductive responsibility cannot bear the weight of coercive state enforcement, the reproductive choices of individuals and communities and the standards underlying them should not for this reason be banished from the realm of public discussion, debate, and even censure. Indeed, a pluralistic democratic social order cannot be morally indifferent to these matters, for some choices, even if they have the backing of the individual's particular community, are clearly morally irresponsible as judged from the point of view of the common moral standards of that society.[28] And while coercion may be an extreme response in these cases, society may be able to foster adherence to its norms of reproductive responsibility in other nonpunitive, noninvasive ways—for example, by offering small but meaningful incentives to individuals to forgo reproduction.

There will be many situations, of course, in which the reproductive choices of individuals fall into a grey area, somewhere between the clearly responsible and the clearly irresponsible. Different interpretations of reproductive responsibility may be at work, no one of which commands widespread social agreement. Here public discussion and debate can be useful, even if this does not lead to agreement on substantive moral values for the society. By listening to what others have to say about their reproductive choices and engaging in constructive dialogue with them on the grounds for these decisions, our respective thinking about reproductive responsibility might change. Or we might find that there are already significant points of convergence between our understandings of these matters. Even if we remain divided in our views of reproductive responsibility, we might at least be better able to articulate the grounds of our respective differences. Though questions about reproductive responsibility can be asked wholly in private, both our personal and communal lives will stand to be significantly enriched if we talk about them together.

NOTES

1. Gen. 1:28.

2. Margaret Polaneczky, Gail Slap, Christine Forke, et al., "Use of Levonorgestrel Implants (Norplant) for Contraception in Adolescent Mothers," NEJM 331: 18 (3 November 1994): 1201–1206. In this study of ninety-eight inner-city mothers, forty-eight chose Norplant and fifty chose the pill. A year and a half later, of the forty-eight on Norplant only one became pregnant, while nineteen of those on the pill (38%) became pregnant.

3. Ellen H. Moskowitz, Bruce Jennings, and Daniel Callahan, "Long-Acting Contraceptives: Ethical Guidance for Policymakers and Health Care Providers," this volume.

4. Three notions are relevant to the issue of blame: excuse, mitigation, and justification. When an act is justified, what is done is something which morality (or law) does not condemn and may even welcome. In this case, there is nothing for which to blame or punish the agent. When an act is excusable, the act itself is morally (or legally) prohibited, but blame or punishment is excluded because of factors which render the action unintentional or involuntary or the agent incapable of choice or self-control. Mitigation presupposes that the individual has acted wrongly and is liable to be blamed or punished. The question is not whether blame or punishment is appropriate, but how severe it should be. See H. L. A. Hart, *Punishment and Responsibility* (New York: Oxford University Press, 1968), 13–17. The section on "Assigning Blame" discusses excusing and mitigating factors, but as we note in the section on "Multiculturalism and Reproductive Responsibility," there are those who argue that cultural differences can preclude moral criticism of reproductive acts themselves.

5. This view is presented and rejected in Bonnie Steinbock and Ron McClamrock, "When Is Birth Unfair to the Child?" *Hastings Center Report* 24 (November–December 1994): 15–21.

6. "Wrongful Life and the Counterfactual Element in Harming," *Social Philosophy and Policy* 4 (1987), 145–178.

7. This is in fact the position John Robertson takes in "Norplant and Irresponsible Reproduction," *Hastings Center Report* 25 (January–February 1995): S23-S26.

8. Thomas Nagel, *The View from Nowhere* (New York: Oxford University Press, 1986).

9. Carol Levine and Nancy N. Dubler, "Uncertain Risks and Bitter Realities: The Reproductive Choices of HIV-infected Women," *Milbank Quarterly* 68, no. 3 (1990): 321–52.

10. Anita Allen, "Moral Multiculturalism, Childbearing, and AIDS," in *HIV, AIDS, and Childbearing: Public Policy, Private Lives,* ed. Ruth Faden and Nancy Kass (New York: Oxford University Press, 1996), 367–407.

11. Levine and Dubler, "Uncertain Risks," 345–46.

12. Stephan A. James, "Reconciling International Human Rights and Cultural Relativism: The Case of Female Circumcision," *Bioethics,* no. 1 (1994): 1–26.

13. Robert M. Cover, *Justice Accused: Antislavery and the Judicial Process* (New Haven: Yale University Press, 1975).

14. Allen, "Moral Multiculturalism," 388.

15. Hans Georg Gadamer, *Truth and Method*, 2nd ed., tr. Joel Weinsheimer and D. G. Marshall (New York: Crossroad, 1989), 302–06. On the problem of translation between cultures, see Alasdair MacIntyre, *Whose Justice? Which Rationality?* (Notre Dame: University of Notre Dame Press, 1988), 370–88.

16. Charles Taylor, *Multiculturalism and "The Politics of Recognition,"* (Princeton: Princeton University Press, 1992), 67, 70.

17. Samuel Fleischacker, *The Ethics of Culture* (Ithaca, N.Y.: Cornell University Press, 1994), 149–199.

18. Michael Walzer provides numerous examples of this "internalist" variety of criticism in *Interpretation and Social Criticism* (Cambridge: Harvard University Press, 1987) and *The Company of Critics: Social Criticism and Political Commitment in the Twentieth Century* (New York: Basic Books, 1988).

19. Allen, "Moral Multiculturalism," 370.

20. Michael Walzer, *Thick and Thin: Moral Argument at Home and Abroad* (Notre Dame: Notre Dame University Press, 1994).

21. Robert K. Fullinwider, "Ethnocentrism and Education in Judgment," *Report from the Institute for Philosophy & Public Policy* 14 (1994): 6–11.

22. Norvin Richards, *Humility* (Philadelphia: Temple University Press, 1992).

23. Amy Gutmann, "The Challenge of Multiculturalism in Political Ethics," *Philosophy & Public Affairs* 22, no.3 (1993): 171–206.

24. Philip J. Hilts, "Implant Easily Surpasses Pill in Averting Teen-Age Pregnancy," *New York Times* (Thursday, November 3, 1994), B14.

25. Anita Allen, "Moral Multiculturalism."

26. Bonnie Steinbock, "The Concept of Coercion and Long-Term Contraceptives," this volume, 62–96.

27. Much depends, however, on the mode of deployment. If such exhortations to refrain from childbearing are targeted solely at teens from poor, urban minority districts, their effect will be highly discriminatory and therefore unjustified. Noncoercive programs must therefore satisfy other criteria of justice such as uniform application.

28. One woman cited by Anita Allen provides an extraordinary example of what we (i.e., the authors) would regard as an irresponsible attitude toward reproduction.

En route to making the point that women who have lost custody of their previous children—e.g., through drug abuse or neglect—often exhibit the greatest desire to reproduce in spite of the 25% risk of transmitting HIV, Professor Allen quotes a woman as saying that ". . . it is better to have an HIV baby than a drug baby because: 'the drug baby, they gonna take away from you,' but the HIV baby you can keep." See "Moral Multiculturalism," 390. One can have enormous sympathy for such a woman, whose very identity might well depend upon her ability to have and keep a child, while still rejecting in the strongest possible terms a value ordering that would place her own needs and happiness above the very life of an HIV-infected child. Prenatal drug addiction and subsequent loss of custody may well represent harms to both child and mother, but we would submit that they both pale in comparison to the lethal harm involved in transmitting HIV, and eventually AIDS, to one's own child.

REBECCA DRESSER

Long-Term Contraceptives in the Criminal Justice System

One week after Norplant was approved by the U.S. Food and Drug Administration, it was incorporated into the sentence imposed on a woman convicted of child abuse. In a criminal justice system beset by inadequate financial resources, large numbers of child abuse and neglect cases, and a longing for easy answers to complex problems, one judge found Norplant a welcome addition to his array of sentencing options. In very short order, a device created to expand women's reproductive freedom was revealed as a potential instrument of state power.

This chapter analyzes the use of long-term contraceptives as punishment. My emphasis is on the practice's ethical and policy dimensions as opposed to the precise constitutional and statutory law issues it raises. Some commentators have argued, perhaps correctly, that contraceptive sentences impermissibly violate constitutional rights to privacy, equality, and bodily integrity.[1] If so, appellate courts will eventually overrule trial judges sentencing women to contraceptives and legislators enacting laws specifically authorizing the practice. It is also possible that appellate courts will strike down judicial orders for contraceptive use on the grounds that such orders fail to meet statutory principles delineating the appropriate scope of probation conditions.[2]

Not all contraceptive sentences will be appealed, however.[3] Moreover, such sentences might survive appellate review in some jurisdictions.[4] If it turns out that the law permits judges to impose long-acting contraceptives as punishment and legislators to enact statutes authorizing such sentences, when, if ever, should they do so? What are the general moral and policy considerations relevant to contraceptive sentencing? By going beyond the narrow legal analysis, I hope to enrich and expand the evaluation of contraceptives in the criminal justice system.

Four Cases

To gain a sense of the subject's scope and complexity, let us first examine a few of the recent court cases in which reproductive restrictions were imposed as punishment. A look at these cases reveals something about the judges' motivations in sentencing and about the situations of the women and children involved. Although defendants convicted of a wide variety of offenses have been ordered or asked to accept sterilization or contraception, the primary target offenses are child abuse and child neglect.[5] As authorities increasingly prosecute women for prenatal child abuse, contraceptive sentencing could affect women convicted of this offense as well.[6] Because Norplant, Depo-Provera, and other long-acting contraceptives are highly effective, less drastic than surgical sterilization, and more easily monitored than other forms of contraception, they are likely to become the punishments of choice whenever lawmakers and judges seek to restrict the reproductive capacity of women offenders. Although three of the cases discussed below involved other forms of reproductive interventions, they serve as models for the kinds of cases in which long-term contraceptives are likely to be invoked in the future.

Decided in 1984, here is an early example of court-ordered contraception as a condition of probation for a woman convicted of child abuse. A jury convicted Ruby Pointer of felony child endangerment. She followed a strict macrobiotic diet, which she applied to her two sons as well. Medical and social services workers warned her about the diet's risk to her children. After one of her sons was hospitalized and removed from her custody, she seized him and fled to Puerto Rico, where she was eventually captured. By this time, both sons were significantly malnourished, and one had suffered permananent neurological impairment.

Ruby Pointer was given a five-year probation term, the children were removed from her custody, and she was ordered to undergo counselling and to refrain from becoming pregnant during the probation period. On appeal, the court struck down the conception prohibition on the grounds that it was unnecessarily intrusive. The appellate court accepted the need to protect future children from *in utero* harm caused by the diet, but believed this need could be addressed by requiring the defendant to have periodic pregnancy tests, to obtain prenatal care for future pregnancies, and to relinquish custody of any future children in apparent danger. The court disregarded the state's contention that local probation officials lacked the resources necessary to furnish the close supervision this less drastic alternative would require.

The unfortunate sequel to this case became public in 1991. Responding to neighbors' complaints about suspected child abuse, police discovered Ruby Pointer with three young daughters aged two, four, and six. The children were malnourished and unable to speak, for they had experienced little contact with the outside world. At least one of the children was born during the earlier probation period, and another was probably conceived during that time.

Apparently, the appellate court's instructions were not fully implemented. In addition, although police and child protective services workers had received other calls about possible beatings occurring in Pointer's apartment, nothing had been done to protect the children despite her prior record.[7]

Tracy Wilder was a seventeen-year-old successful high school student. In 1990, she became pregnant, but told no one about it. After her mother brought her to an emergency room for treatment of abdominal pains, Wilder gave birth to a child in the hospital bathroom. She then smothered the child and put her in the wastebasket. She was charged with second-degree murder, which carried a possible prison term of twelve to twenty-two years. She agreed to plead guilty to the less serious offense of manslaughter and in turn received a sentence of two years in prison and ten years of probation, conditioned on her completion of high school, acceptance of psychological and contraceptive counseling, and use of contraceptives during the probation period.

The American Civil Liberties Union and the Family Research Council (an antiabortion group) opposed the contraceptive provision of this plea agreement. But Wilder rejected the ACLU's offer of free representation to challenge the condition. Wilder's attorney reported that his client saw the contraception condition as an alternative to spending many years in prison. As her legal representative, his paramount concern was his client's freedom from physical confinement, which he did not want to jeopardize by filing an appeal: "I place a higher value on freedom than being concerned about a probation condition. I'm more concerned about getting this girl back home than the social ramifications for other people."[8]

Darlene Johnson was the first woman ordered to receive Norplant as a condition of probation. In 1991, Johnson, who was pregnant with her fifth child, was convicted of corporal child abuse. The children had been severely beaten with an electric cord and belt buckle, which produced widespread and significant bruises and scars.

Johnson was eligible for a six-year prison term, in part due to her prior criminal record, which consisted primarily of property-related offenses. Instead, Judge Howard Broadman sentenced her to three years of probation. She was to spend one year in jail, primarily so that her conduct during pregnancy could be monitored to prevent alcohol, drug, and tobacco use. She was also ordered to participate in psychological counselling and parenting skills classes. Last, Broadman conditioned the probation order on Johnson's willingness to use Norplant for the probationary period that followed the birth of her child. At the sentencing hearing she agreed to the probation condition, but her consent was based on the judge's sketchy description of the device, which omitted any information on medical risks. A week later, her attorney moved to modify the condition, partially because Johnson had high blood pressure and diabetes, both of which enhance the device's risks. The judge denied the motion, and an appeal was filed. Before it could be argued, however, Johnson's probation was revoked because she tested positive for cocaine use on three occasions. In the meantime, Broadman removed himself from the case after an abortion opponent fired a gun at him in anger over the attempt to interfere with procreation. The judge who replaced Broadman sent Johnson to prison for five years.[9]

Last is an early 1993 Tennessee case involving Barbara and Ronald Gross, a married couple who pleaded guilty to attempted aggravated sexual battering of two of their children. The judge offered them two alternatives: (1) five-year prison terms for each defendant, or (2) ten years probation for each of them on condition that the *woman* consent to tubal ligation. No reproductive constraints were imposed on Ronald Gross as conditions of the latter option. Barbara Gross had herself been molested as a child and her own father was believed to be the father of her eldest child. She had also been diagnosed as having a schizoaffective disorder and was believed to be mentally retarded. There were four children in the family, and she was pregnant with the fifth when she was sentenced, though the state had moved to terminate the couple's parental rights. The judge deemed sterilization unnecessary for Ronald Gross because he was "a faithful husband" and would pose no risk to future children if his wife were sterilized. Although she was of questionable competency and was given no information on the sterilization procedure, the court accepted Barbara Gross's consent to the surgery.[10]

The Social Context

These cases provoke in us a variety of responses. To understand and evaluate both the judges' conduct and our reactions to it, it is worthwhile to consider a few specific elements of the social context in which the contraceptive sentences are situated.

Two background conditions are influencing the judges sentencing women to reproductive restrictions. One is the judges' growing frustration and disillusionment with the lack of effect traditional punishment approaches appear to have on persons who harm their children, particularly when substance abuse is involved. Judges have publicly lamented the "exploding numbers" of abuse and neglect cases and expressed frustration at their inability to address the problem.[11] Their concern extends to the increasing number of children born affected by their mothers' drug use.[12] It is evident in the move to criminalize gestational abuse; including birth control in the sentences imposed on such offenders seems logically related to the approach. It is undeniable that judges today see many children who bear the burdens of their parents' irresponsible behavior. The judges' legitimate quest to protect children more effectively makes long-term contraceptives seem an attractive, easily monitored means to avoid adding more stress and more potential victims to the offenders' troubled life situations.[13] Another force driving contraceptive sentencing is the increased support for what have been labeled "intermediate" or "alternative" punishments. Spurred by the existence of overcrowded prisons, ineffective probation services, and academic challenges to the assumption that punishment necessarily involves incarceration, policymakers have begun to advocate more extensive use of measures such as "intensive supervision" probation (including house arrest, electronic monitoring of the offender's location, and other stringent restrictions on the offender's physical freedom in the community), relatively severe fines calibrated to the offender's earning capacity, closely supervised and enforced community service, and rigorous drug and alcohol treatment programs. These sanctions are considered most suitable for persons convicted of serious crimes who would be eligible for moderate prison terms, but would not pose a serious danger to the community with proper restriction. Intermediate sanctions are not designed to dispense with the retributive elements of punishment. Instead, they are designed to impose burdens and limit autonomy by means other than incarceration. Advocates of this approach argue that intermediate punishment should be roughly equivalent in severity to the prison term to which the offender could otherwise be subjected.[14]

The negative reactions to contraceptive sentencing also have roots in broader social concerns. For example, feminist commentary almost uniformly condemns the incorporation of contraception into a criminal sentence on the grounds that the state should be prohibited from interfering with a woman's reproductive freedom and physical integrity in this manner. It is feared that contraceptive punishment is simply the most recent surfacing of the state's recurring effort to gain control over women's, particularly poor African-American and Latina women's, fertility. Feminists have expressed considerable worry about the slippery slope effects of this measure, predicting that if reproductive autonomy may be infringed in the criminal system, other types of state interference will follow.[15]

There are additional contextual sources of the critical reaction to contraception as punishment, including pro-life and civil liberties groups' opposition to the practice, general discontent with the criminal justice system's seeming failure to control crime and its ill effects, basic disagreement over the role of free will versus economic, social, and biological factors in causing criminal behavior, and a sense that society ought to offer more affirmative programs to assist members of disadvantaged groups disproportionately represented in jails, prisons, and other punishment institutions. It is helpful to keep these various social pressures in mind in attempting to formulate a principled stance on contraceptive punishment.

Is Contraception Justified Punishment?

To evaluate the merits and drawbacks of contraception as punishment, one must consider why any sort of punishment may be imposed on persons convicted of crime. Punishment is usually justified as a means of advancing four goals: retribution, deterrence, incapacitation, and rehabilitation. What follows is a brief description of each of these punishment rationales and a discussion of the degree to which orders to use contraceptives are compatible with these aims.

Retributive principles have the strongest influence on contemporary punishment theory and practice. According to retributive theory, persons who commit crimes deserve punishment. Because such individuals have harmed their victim's and community's welfare, the state is in turn entitled to subject them to the burdens and stigma of punishment. On the retributive model, punishment must be proportionate to the offender's level of culpability and to the harm produced by the criminal behavior. Serious crimes merit heavy sanctions; less serious offenses call for more moderate punitive measures.

Do contraceptive sentences fit the retributive model of punishment? The retributivist would be receptive to such sentences as long as they met the general requirements for punishment. The retributivist would demand rough equivalence between any intermediate sanctions proposed for a particular offense and the prison term that could otherwise be imposed. The intrusions on autonomy and the experiential burdens of the two types of punishment must be similar. Meeting this demand would require sentencing officials to evaluate the nature of the contraceptive measure—its benefits and burdens (including the length of required use)—and then to compare it to other sanctions deemed suitable for the defendant's specific offense. To qualify as a suitable punishment for murder or other severe forms of child abuse, the retributivist would probably demand at a minimum that contraceptive sentencing be supplemented by other significant burdens and restrictions. On the other hand, the retributivist might well reject the imposition of contraceptive sentences in less serious abuse and neglect cases.[16]

The remaining three justifications for punishment—deterrence, incapacitation, and rehabilitation—all seek to achieve future societal benefits by imposing criminal sanctions. Their overall aim is crime reduction, which may be promoted through actions directed at the individual offender or the broader society. Deterrence operates at both these levels. Specific deterrence focuses on preventing the punished individual from committing future crimes. Punishment is inflicted to impress on the offender the risks accompanying a decision to engage in wrongdoing. According to the specific deterrence model, sentences should be calibrated to the offender's individual characteristics and situation. Defendants who refuse to acknowledge responsibility, have prior criminal records, or evidence other characteristics suggesting that they will be relatively less responsive to corrective measures will receive heavier sentences than those who appear more easily deterred.

General deterrence is aimed at the broader community. Punishment of convicted individuals is justified on the grounds that it will discourage other members of society who might be tempted to engage in criminal behavior. Punishment changes the incentive system to reduce the potential advantages of engaging in criminal behavior. Would-be wrongdoers are more likely to abandon their plans for criminal activity if they recognize that they too could experience the burdensome restrictions imposed on convicted offenders.[17]

Deterrence strategy could be influencing some judges to propose contraceptive sentences. When they encounter a woman whose parenting behavior appears persistently irresponsible, they might see court-ordered contraception as a burden that could effectively discourage her from such behavior in the future. Yet it is difficult to understand why enforced contraception would be a particularly effective deterrent in most cases. It is more likely that judges have in mind general deterrence when they invoke contraceptive sentences. The judges may intend through their actions to notify the public that they are serious about discouraging child abuse and neglect and are ready to resort to strong measures to do so.[18] If general deterrence is indeed their aim, the ethical and policy questions concern whether contraceptive sentences will actually discourage potential offenders and whether the intrusion on the defendant's physical integrity and reproductive autonomy is justified to promote the greater good.

Incapacitation is another forward-looking punishment aim. Incapacitative punishment is designed to prevent future crime by removing the offender's opportunity to repeat her behavior. People in prison are removed from most of their potential victims and the means necessary to commit many crimes. Certain probation conditions have incapacitation as their goal—for example, house arrest, electronic monitoring, and other forms of close supervision. Incapacitation simply puts physical and other barriers in the way of persons who seek to persist in their criminal activities.[19]

Judges have sometimes explicitly invoked the goal of incapacitation to justify contraceptive sentences. They have expressed hope that a defendant's contraceptive use will prevent her from injuring future children. For example, in sentencing Darlene Johnson, Judge Broadman remarked: "It is . . . certainly in any unconceived child's interest that [the defendant] not have any more children until she is mentally and emotionally prepared to do so."[20] Preventing women from conceiving substantially reduces their access to new victims during the punishment period. When this measure is combined with removal of existing children from the home, the probation conditions create an effective obstacle to commission of future crimes.

Yet the underlying logic of the incapacitative rationale for contraceptive sentencing can be challenged on two grounds. First, this justification depends on the philosophically sticky idea that potential future children can be protected by preventing their very existence.[21] Second, it extends legal protection and concern to unborn—indeed, to unconceived—children. Although there are a few other areas in which the law arguably seeks to confer such protection, such as through permitting sterilization of mentally disabled adults and prohibiting the practice of surrogate motherhood, these laws are controversial and justifiable on alternative grounds as well.[22] A further issue concerns whether the hoped-for incapacitative effect could be achieved by more acceptable means. A few appellate courts reviewing contraceptive sentences have accepted the contention that contraceptive sentences are reasonably related to the goal of preventing future child abuse and neglect, but have rejected the sentences on the grounds that this goal could be achieved through less intrusive means.[23]

Rehabilitation is the final of the four traditional punishment goals. Rehabilitative punishment seeks to change the individual offender into a law-abiding citizen through enhancing her chances for successful community life. Typical rehabilitative measures are education, job training, and counselling. Although at one time rehabilitation was the dominant goal of the United States penal system, in the last quarter-century its appeal has diminished. The current disillusionment with rehabilitation is based on the lack of persuasive evidence that rehabilitative programs promote individual change, and on the belief that rehabilitative programs were premised on ethically questionable principles— namely, that individual defendants are "beings to be manipulated and controlled" by the state.[24] This is not to suggest that rehabilitative efforts have been completely abandoned, but simply to note their relatively minor role in contemporary punishment policy.

Contraceptive sentences have been justified as rehabilitative. For example, Howard Broadman claimed a rehabilitative intent when he sentenced Darlene Johnson to three years of Norplant use:

Invading a human being's body is a big step. But locking somebody up in prison is also a big step. Clearly, I could just have locked her up for four years, but I thought it would be better to try to keep the family together, to see if she could get her act together. I thought that not having more children in the next three years would help in her potential rehabilitation.[25]

Judge Broadman's rehabilitation claim rests on the belief that preventing future births would reduce stress and other impediments to Darlene Johnson's becoming a nonabusive parent. There is some evidence that large family size is one factor associated with maternal violence toward children, although no direct relationship has been established.[26] Yet parenting classes, counselling, and similar measures also offer less extreme alternatives to promote a defendant's rehabilitation.[27]

No form of punishment is perfectly justified in light of traditional punishment goals. Contraceptive sentencing joins other contemporary punishment practices in offering a possible means of advancing some of these goals. Thus contraceptive sentencing cannot be definitively ruled out as inconsistent with punishment theory. Thorough evaluation of contraceptive sentencing demands attention to two additional dimensions of the practice, however. These are its coercive elements and its likely disproportionate effect on low-income women, especially low-income women of color.

Coercion and Disproportionate Impacts

Contraceptive sentencing occurs in a system which is itself highly coercive. A fundamental principle of the criminal justice system is that the state is morally authorized—indeed, morally required—to deprive convicted offenders of substantial freedom and experiential comfort. All forms of punishment are coercively imposed. Offenders in most cases are given little choice of how they will be punished. If probation is proposed, it may be conditioned on the defendant's acceptance of numerous restrictions and infringements of her usual rights and liberties. It is in this coercive context, then, that the coercion entailed in contraceptive sentencing must be evaluated.

The most recent instances of contraceptive sentencing involved conditions of probation imposed on convicted defendants. In these cases, there was an alternative to court-ordered birth control available to the defendant: the prison sentence she would otherwise have received.[28] Does this availability of another choice make defendant's agreement to court-ordered contraception sufficiently voluntary to survive moral scrutiny? This complex question lies at the heart of the dispute over the permissibility of contraceptive sentencing. One response is that the contraceptive proposal puts the defendant in a coercive situation, "given that many people will agree to almost anything to avoid doing time."[29] Yet it is also possible to argue that the proposal improves the defendant's situation. On this view, a prohibition on contraceptive sentences would "wrongfully deprive some women of a legitimate option."[30]

Is a judge's proposal to order probation conditioned on a convicted defendant's use of a long-acting contraceptive a freedom-enhancing offer or a freedom-restricting threat? According to Alan Wertheimer's coercion analysis, a proposal qualifies as an offer if declining it would leave the choosing individual no worse off than she is in her current, or baseline, situation. On the other hand, declining a coercive threat leaves a person worse off than she was in her baseline situation.[31] In this framework, contraceptive sentencing could qualify as a noncoercive offer since the typical convicted woman's baseline situation includes the prospect of a prison term. Declining the probation condition thus leaves her no worse off than she was in her baseline situation.

But the calculation is a bit trickier than this because the very availability of contraceptive sentencing could negatively influence the specific defendant's baseline situation. If the contraceptive option were unavailable, what sentence would the judge actually impose on this defendant? Would it be another variation of probation with less intrusive conditions? If it would be a prison term, what would be the length, location, and nature of the defendant's incarceration? Would it be for a short time in a relatively tolerable setting? Would the defendant be offered educational or other benefits during the time she was incarcerated?

The answers to these counterfactual questions are somewhat elusive because it is difficult for the observer, and perhaps even the judges themselves, to determine what a defendant's sentence would have been if court-ordered contraception were unavailable. The danger is that the sentence would have involved fewer burdens than either of the two options now facing the defendant—probation conditioned on contraceptive use or a burdensome period of incarceration. If so, the very availability of easily monitored long-term contraceptives leaves such women worse off than they were in their baseline situations.

Contraceptive sentences could thus reduce the overall freedom of at least some women convicted of child abuse and neglect. At the same time, such sentences could enhance the freedom of offenders whose baseline situations include a substantial and burdensome prison term. The problem comes in identifying which category an individual woman occupies. Some guidance could come through examining the noncontraceptive sentences imposed on persons convicted of similar offenses. If a woman is presented with the option of probation with contraceptive use or an alternative punishment that resembles what is typically given to defendants in her circumstances, then the contraceptive condition could reasonably be viewed as a freedom-enhancing offer.[32]

But perhaps it is something about the nature of the contraceptive probation condition that creates special concern about its coercive potential. The possibility that defendants would experience unusual pressure in deciding whether or not to use Norplant is troubling on two scores. Subjecting women to this situation seems to contradict the strong legal and ethical support for protecting individual autonomy in medical and reproductive decision making. Because of the physical intrusions and health risks that accompany interventions such as long-acting contraceptives, our policies normally require the state to refrain from involvement in medical decision making. A similar stance is taken toward decisions about procreation and the family because of the intensely personal nature of these matters. The explicit entry of fertility control into the realm of punishment seems to conflict with these general principles.

At the same time, prison terms and conditions of probation typically impose restrictions on many of the rights and freedoms enjoyed by ordinary citizens. Convicted defendants often consent to give up legally protected rights to avoid going to prison. These may include restrictions on their religious, speech, assembly, association (including contact with family members), and privacy rights. Probation conditions may also include physically invasive measures, such as treatment for mental illness or substance abuse and testing for sexually transmitted disease or controlled substance use.[33] In this framework, it seems, if the consent of a defendant such as Darlene Johnson "was vitiated by the coercive influence of her desire to avoid prison, the validity of all probation conditions might be questioned."[34] Yet appellate courts have failed to reject as overly coercive the convicted person's consent to many highly restrictive probation conditions.

So the harsh context of the criminal justice system weakens the claim that contraceptive sentencing is extraordinarily coercive. Within this context, it is not unreasonable to label such sentencing freedom-enhancing for at least some women. Moreover, the fact that such defendants consent to infringements on their fundamental personal rights fails to distinguish contraceptive sentences from other probation conditions. The options presented to women in these cases are not distinctively different from those faced by other criminal offenders.

The disproportionate gender, race, and class effects of contraceptive sentencing constitute a second reason to be disturbed about the practice, however. None of the most recent cases involved male defendants convicted of child abuse or neglect, although judges have in the past included among probation conditions imposed on men orders to curtail reproduction or sexual activity.[35] The disparate impact is partially attributable to the absence of an effective, enforceable male contraceptive. At present, contraceptive sentencing for men is limited to primarily symbolic exhortations or the drastic remedy of permanent sterilization. Male sex offenders have received Depo-Provera and other antiandrogens to reduce inappropriate sexual desires, but the sole appellate decision addressing the permissibility of this intervention as a probation condition rejected it on the grounds that the medical community at that time had not accepted the agent for use in suppressing the male sex drive.[36]

Feminist concern about potential gender bias in contraceptive sentencing is valid. The emergence of long-term implantable and injectable contraceptives supplies added reason for concern because they are effective, easily monitored, and can be used only in women. As such, these methods could easily become vehicles for exercising control over women's lives in a variety of settings. If long-term contraceptives are adopted in the criminal justice system, their attractiveness as a means to promote or impose state policy in other areas could increase. Especially when considered in tandem with other state efforts to control women's reproductive freedom—including punishment of drug use in pregnancy, court-ordered Caesarean sections, and stricter regulation of abortion—the slippery slope and symbolic effects of contraceptive sentences are real and should not be dismissed.[37]

Similar concerns exist regarding the kinds of women who are likely to be the subjects of contraceptive sentencing. I have no doubt that they will be overwhelmingly poor, and many will be women of color. Poor women are more likely than others to be reported for prenatal drug use.[38] Because they tend to have more personal contact with government agencies than people in higher economic classes, their child-rearing practices are subject to greater scrutiny by outsiders.[39] When neglect or abuse is discovered, officials may more readily set prosecutions in motion when they would resort to less punitive measures if parents were middle- or upper-class.[40] Our nation also has a history of promoting sterilization of low-income women and women of color to advance eugenic, racist, and population control goals. Such motives could play a covert role in decisions to propose long-acting contraceptives as probation conditions for women belonging to these groups.[41]

Contraceptive Sentencing: A Proposal

Contraceptive sentencing has an unclear legal future. Appellate courts may reject the practice on statutory or constitutional grounds. Yet some courts may affirm orders for contraceptive use. Moreover, some women may follow

Tracey Wilder in choosing to accept their contraceptive sentences. In short, contraceptive sentences may be available as punishment options. How should persons concerned about misuse approach this situation? One strategy would be to try to persuade judges and legislators that contraceptives should never be part of criminal sentences because of the potential for coercion; disproportionate gender, race, and class impacts; and danger to women's reproductive and medical autonomy. This may be the wisest course given the danger that widespread abuse could accompany any resort to contraceptive sentencing.

Yet I hesitate to endorse this option because I can imagine some cases in which contraceptive use would be a legitimate component of a sentence. For some women, contraceptive use might be a genuinely preferred and effective option to the possible alternative controls on their freedom. It seems unfair to such women and to the broader community to reject this option because of the risks it could pose to others. Banning contraceptives from the realm of punishment would leave convicted women to face prison terms and other traditionally accepted forms of punishment, which could be more burdensome and less effective in reducing the possibility of future criminality. Moreover, banning long-term contraceptives would not do anything to improve the difficulties these women and their children now face. The unsatisfactory status quo would remain intact.

One way to reconcile the competing concerns would be to adopt the following principle: whenever long-acting contraceptives are proposed as a probation condition, judges must also present to the defendant at least one nonincarcerative alternative sentence. If the defendant was convicted of an offense that would not ordinarily call for a prison term, then she should be given two alternatives: one including contraceptives as a probation condition, and one including a set of noncontraceptive probation conditions customarily applied to defendants in her situation.[42] If individuals convicted of the offense are eligible for a prison term, and the judge believes that probation with contraceptive use would be an appropriate alternative, the judge would be obligated to make three proposals: probation with contraceptive use, an alternative set of probation conditions, and the prison term the defendant would normally have to serve. Adherence to this principle would remove some of the pressure a defendant might feel to compromise her medical or reproductive preferences for the sake of avoiding confinement in a correctional institution.

The proposal fails to offer a perfect resolution. It may deter some judges from offering any probationary sentence at all. Yet by supplying a constraint that would discourage liberal judicial use of contraceptive sentencing, the proposal reduces the ethically troubling aspects of the practice. It makes long-acting contraceptives a less significant component in the criminal justice system's response to women convicted of child abuse and neglect and gives the defendant an opportunity to avoid these interventions without completely forgoing the probation option.

Contraceptive sentencing can have only the most minimal impact on the incidence of child abuse and neglect. I close with a reminder of all the other measures that would be incorporated into a governmental system that was truly serious about protecting children from this form of harm. Such a system would include a probation office with enough employees to implement the conditions of probation ordered by courts. It would include high-quality counselling and education for overwhelmed parents. It would include help for substance-abusing parents and job and educational training for those in need of employment. It would include a child protective services system that responded promptly to reports of abuse or neglect. It would include teacher training programs on detection of children at risk. It would include regular health care by professionals familiar with the signs of abuse and neglect. It would include good prenatal care and full family planning services for poor women.

We ought to direct our energies to developing and supporting a system like this. Seizing on long-term contraceptives and other punitive measures to solve the problems of abused and neglected children is shortsighted at best. We must not allow this strategy to divert our country from the real and pressing obligations we have to improve the lives of these children and those who care for them in very difficult circumstances.

NOTES

1. See, for example, Kristyn Walker, "Judicial Control of Reproductive Freedom: The Use of Norplant as a Condition of Probation," *Iowa Law Review* 78, no. 3 (1993): 779–812; Julie Mertus and Simon Heller, "Norplant Meets the New Eugenicists: The Impermissibility of Coerced Contraception," *Saint Louis University Public Law Review* 11, no. 2 (1992): 359–83.

2. In general, the laws governing probation require that all conditions contained in a probationary sentence be reasonably related to the permissible goals of probation. The requirement has been interpreted in a variety of ways, with some courts applying it more stringently than others. See Stacey Arthur, "The Norplant Prescription: Birth Control, Woman Control, or Crime Control?" *UCLA Law Review* 40, no. 1 (1992): 1–101.

3. See Guttmacher Institute, "Update—Recent Court Actions on Forced Norplant Use," *Norplant: Opportunities and Perils for Low-Income Women,* no. 2 (July 1993): 5–6.

4. One author who believes that Norplant probation conditions are legally permissible under certain circumstances is Michael Flannery, "Norplant: The New Scarlet Letter?" *Journal of Contemporary Health Law and Policy* 8 (Spring 1992): 201–26.

5. Contraceptive probation conditions imposed on defendants convicted of crimes unrelated to harming children are probably legally invalid under statutes requiring that probation conditions be reasonably related to preventing or discouraging an offender from engaging in similar criminal behavior in the future. See Arthur, "Norplant Prescription," 51–3.

6. See Flannery, "New Scarlet Letter," 210. During the past two years, a number of state legislative bills were introduced providing for the use of Norplant in punishment. Most were directed against women convicted of prenatal drug abuse; none have been enacted into law. For summaries of some of these bills, see Mertus and Heller, "Norplant Meets the New Eugenicists," 363; Guttmacher Institute, "Update—Proposed State Legislation to Provide or Mandate Use of Norplant," *Norplant: Opportunities and Perils for Low-Income Women,* no. 1 (December 1992): 3–4; Center for Reproductive Law and Policy, "In the States," *Reproductive Freedom News* 2, no. 3 (5 February 1993): 7. A recently enacted Illinois statute prohibits judges from mandating any form of birth control as part of a criminal sentence. Center for Reproductive Law and Policy, "In the States," *Reproductive Freedom News* 2, no. 16 (25 February 1993): 6.

7. For description and discussion of this case, see Arthur, "Norplant Prescription," 42–3, 70–5; Mertus and Heller, "Norplant Meets the New Eugenicists," 365–6; Flannery, "New Scarlet Letter," 211.

8. Quoted in Felicity Barringer, "Sentence for Killing Newborn: Jail Term, Then Birth Control," *New York Times*, 18 November 1990, pp. A1, A21. Details of the case are also provided in Arthur, "Norplant Prescription," 13–5.

9. The case is described in detail in Walker, "Norplant as Probation," 789–91; Arthur, "Norplant Prescription," 15–19; Flannery, "New Scarlet Letter," 211–13; Mertus and Heller, "Norplant Meets the New Eugenicists," pp. 364–67. Since this case, there have been several others in which judges proposed Norplant as part of a criminal sentence. See Madeline Henley, "The Creation and Perpetuation of the Mother/Body Myth," *Buffalo Law Review* 41, no. 2 (1993): 703–77.

10. See *Tennessee v. Gross,* Nos. 19507 and 19508, Criminal Court, Washington County, Tennessee, Transcript of Probation Hearing January 15, 1993; State of Tennessee Department of Correction, Investigation Report on Barbara Gross, December 3, 1992; "Woman Who Molested Sons Agrees to Sterilization," *New York Times*, 31 January 1993, A29; "Sterilization—and Unfit Mothers," *New York Times*, 12 February 1993, A32.

11. See Arthur, "Norplant Prescription," 24–27.

12. See Flannery, "New Scarlet Letter," 210.

13. See also Cheri Pies, "Creating Ethical Reproductive Health Care Policy," *Education Programs Associates* (1993): 29–31, which reports similar opinions voiced by health care professionals and policymakers.

14. For general discussions of intermediate sanctions, see Norval Morris and Michael Tonry, *Between Prison and Probation* (New York: Oxford University Press, 1990); Andrew von Hirsch, "Community Punishments," in *Principled Sentencing*, ed. Andrew von Hirsch and Andrew Ashworth (Boston: Northeastern University Press, 1992) 325–32; Andrew von Hirsch, Martin Wasik, and Judith Greene, "Scaling Community Punishments," in *Principled Sentencing*, 368–88. The judge who sentenced Darlene Johnson has reportedly sentenced other defendants to house arrest, to Antabuse (to combat a defendant's alcoholism), and to court-ordered "donation" of personal property to charity. See note 10, Flannery, "New Scarlet Letter."

15. See Arthur, "Norplant Prescription," 22–24; Mertus and Heller, "Norplant Meets the New Eugenicists," 368–71.

16. For a summary of the retributive rationale for punishment, see Andrew Ashworth, "Desert," in *Principled Sentencing*, 181–87. For an analysis of intermediate punishments and the retributive rationale, see Morris and Tonry, *Between Prison and Probation*, 84–108.

17. For a summary of general and specific deterrence issues, see Andrew Ashworth, "Deterrence," in *Principled Sentencing*, 53–60.

18. Contraceptive sentencing is endorsed on general deterrence grounds in Thomas Bartrum, "Birth Control as a Condition of Probation—A New Weapon in the War Against Child Abuse," *Kentucky Law Journal* 80, no. 4 (1991–92): 1037–53.

19. For discussions of incapacitation, see Andrew von Hirsch, "Incapacitation," in *Principled Sentencing*, 101–08; Morris and Tonry, *Between Prison and Probation*, 13–14, 180–86, 212–18.

20. Michael Lev, "Judge Firm on Forced Contraception," *New York Times*, 11 January 1991, A12.

21. See John Robertson, "Norplant and Irresponsible Reproduction," this volume.

22. See Arthur, "Norplant Prescription," 47–48.

23. See Arthur, "Norplant Prescription," 56–59, 66–67; American Medical Association Board of Trustees, "Requirements or Incentives by Government for the Use of Long-Acting Contraceptives," *JAMA* 267 (1 April 1992): 1818–21.

24. See Andrew von Hirsch, "Rehabilitation," in *Principled Sentencing*, 1–6, 3.

25. Quoted in Arthur, "Norplant Prescription," note 231.

26. Melissa Burke, "The Constitutionality of the Use of the Norplant Contraceptive Device as a Condition of Punishment," *Hastings Constitutional Law Quarterly* 20, no. 1 (1992): 207–46, 229–30.

27. See Mertus and Heller, "Norplant Meets the New Eugenicists," 374–76; AMA Board of Trustees, "Requirements or Incentives by Government," 1819.

28. See AMA Board of Trustees, "Requirements or Incentives by Government," 1820.

29. Mary Cantwell, "Coercion and Contraception," *New York Times*, 27 January 1991, A16.

30. John MacKenzie, "Whose Choice Is It, Anyway?," *New York Times*, 28 January 1991, A16.

31. See Alan Wertheimer, *Coercion* (Princeton: Princeton University Press, 1987), 202–221.

32. There is general concern that the availability of intermediate sanctions could have a so-called "net-widening" effect, resulting in more severe treatment of defendants who would otherwise have received less restrictive probation conditions. For a proposal addressed to avoiding this outcome, see Andrew von Hirsch, Martin Wasik, and Judith Greene, "Scaling Community Punishments," in *Principled Sentencing*, 368–388.

33. See Morris and Tonry, *Between Prison and Probation*, 186–207; Arthur, "Norplant Prescription," 60–65.

34. Arthur, "Norplant Prescription," 98.

35. See Arthur, "Norplant Prescription," note 32; Mertus and Heller, "Norplant Meets the New Eugenicists," note 98.

36. *People v. Gauntlett,* 134 Mich. App. 737, 352 N.W.2d 310, modified, 353 N.W.2d 463 (1984). See also AMA Trustees, "Requirements or Incentives by Government," 1820.

37. See Arthur, "Norplant Prescription," 22–24; Pies, "Creating Ethical Reproductive Policy," 29–32. Both articles express these concerns.

38. See Ira Chasnoff, Harvey Landress, and Mark Barrett, "The Prevalence of Illicit Drug or Alcohol Use During Pregnancy and Discrepancies in Mandatory Reporting in Pinellas County, Florida," *NEJM* 322, no. 17 (1990): 1202–06.

39. See Dorothy Roberts, "Punishing Drug Addicts Who Have Babies: Women of Color, Equality, and the Right of Privacy," *Harvard Law Review* 104, no. 7 (1991): 1419–81, 1432–33; AMA Board of Trustees, "Requirements or Incentives by Government," 1820.

40. AMA Board of Trustees, "Requirements or Incentives by Government," 1820.

41. See Mertus and Heller, "Norplant Meets the New Eugenicists," 376–83; Roberts, "Punishing Drug Addicts," 1442–44; Walker, "Norplant as Probation," 807–10.

42. The usual legal standards for disclosure of the device's risks and benefits would also have to be met before a defendant's agreement to use Norplant could be accepted.

HILDE LINDEMANN NELSON AND JAMES LINDEMANN NELSON

Other "Isms" Aren't Enough: Feminism, Social Policy, and Long-Acting Contraception

Does feminism provide special, perhaps crucial resources for exploring the ethics of using long-acting contraceptives to shape social policy? At first blush, it might seem that this is a question that answers itself with a resounding yes. If feminism *doesn't* have something distinctively important to say about social policies that so unmistakably target women qua women as do those involving Norplant, Depo-Provera, or IUDs, one might well wonder what the fuss has been about.

On second glance, however, some complexities start to emerge. The first response risks too quickly running together two interrelated but distinct streams of feminist practice, which we will call "feminism as critique" and "feminism as theory." When questions about social policy concerning interventions into female bodies arise, the relevance of feminism as critique, characterized by its vigilance for *defending* the interests of women, should be plain. But the contribution of feminism as theory—at least that portion which might very roughly be described as vigilance in *discerning* the interests of women— is not so immediately apparent. Showing the significance of feminist theory for any responsible exploration of social policies involving long-term contraception will be the central task of this chapter.

In sketch, we will try to answer certain kinds of skepticism about the distinctiveness of feminist theory's contribution to moral thinking in general; along the way, we describe two sorts of difficulties any feminist theorizing encounters in its relationship to other, received theories. We will then argue that feminist theory can indeed make a crucial contribution to responsible decision making about uses of long-term contraceptives in the realm of social policy, offering analyses of their use within the criminal justice system and of policy responses to teenage pregnancy as cases in point. While concerns that emerge with particular clarity and force from feminist theorizing may not be able on their own to resolve these issues decisively, we hope to show that the absence of such theorizing leaves certain social myopias uncorrected, which in turn increases the likelihood that irresponsible policy will be produced.

Feminism as Critique and Feminism as Theory

The core idea of feminism, its basic political and moral insight, can be succinctly stated: women have received unfair, disrespectful, and harmful treatment, substantial in both quantity and degree, in virtue of their being women; this state of affairs is seriously wrong and must be ended.[1] Feminism as critique can be thought of as a series of strategies for disrupting business as usual by calling attention to the ways in which women have been treated unfairly, disrespectfully, and harmfully, and for attempting to change the practices that contribute to this sorry situation. Forcing women to use Norplant as a condition for receiving welfare payments—to take but one proposed social policy use of long-acting contraceptives—clearly calls out for this kind of attention: does such a social practice hurt or wrong women or not? Will its employment make the world a fairer and better place for women or not?

Challenging blatant abuses of women is immensely significant because despite being blatant, they have also been ubiquitous and tenacious in human societies. But precisely because—at least when they've been brought to light in ways that confound efforts to obscure or deny them—those abuses are so blatant, virtually any reasonable moral perspective must condemn them. It doesn't require highly sophisticated theory to see that rape is outrageous or that expecting women to do the same work as men for less compensation is seriously unfair. Some of the contemplated social policy uses of long-acting contraceptives—say, implanting Norplant without supplying the means for its withdrawal—are similarly open to critique by anyone of good will and a clear head. But not all practices that harm or wrong women wear their depravity on their sleeve—including, possibly, some proposed policies regarding long-acting contraceptives. Here, feminism's task goes beyond critique to the construction of a woman-centered conceptual framework that permits a keener discernment of the policy's oppressiveness.

Consider offering Norplant as a condition of probation for women convicted of mistreating their children, for example. A very reasonable case can be mounted that the Norplant offer would be both liberty-enhancing for the woman involved—since it allows her to avoid prison—and welfare-enhancing for the children for whom she cares, since she will not be burdened with further pressures of a kind she apparently finds hard to handle well. A practice of this kind is not, even to feminist-informed sensibilities, a virtually unmistakable instance of abuse. Rather, it presents itself as an apparent dilemma. Any exercise of the state's police power that specifically targets women is *prima facie* suspicious in a misogynist society. But serious moral arguments could be presented in favor of offering Norplant *as an option* to women convicted of child abuse.[2]

If such social policy uses of long-term contraceptives are wrong, it will take something on the order of disciplined, perceptive, articulated moral thinking to show this—that is, it will require something that might well be called a theory. The question then becomes whether feminism has anything particularly important to add when it comes to this task—the construction of a moral perspective that is rationally defensible, enlightening with respect to quandaries of this sort, and distinctive in method.

The Distinctiveness of Feminist Theory

While our opening distinction between feminism as critique and feminism as theory is useful in generating a sense of the problem we confront here, it is also somewhat overstated: feminist theory grows out of feminist critique and nourishes it in turn. Among the ways women have been wronged and harmed in human societies is that they have largely been excluded from theory building itself; they have found it very difficult to be admitted to the company of those whose insights contributed to the intellectual constructs with which we understand our world and act within it.[3] As a consequence, our very awareness of the ways in which women have been wronged are blunt and insensitive.

The core insight of feminism as theory can be put as succinctly as that of feminism simpliciter: women's experiences of the world have been dismissed or downplayed in humankind's efforts to understand reality, and this should cease. On very general methodological grounds, then, it should be clear that adding a perspective so long missing from human theorizing—namely, one that takes women's experiences seriously—will enlarge and enhance our thinking. Just as any viable ethical view will condemn rape, so too any reasonable epistemological view ought to admit the experiences of women. Having done so, we will be in a much better position to assess what is really at stake for women (and for everyone) as we consider policy alternatives regarding long-acting contraceptives, among many others.

But all is not rosy in the feminist-theoretic garden once this is acknowledged. Determining what it is to "admit the experiences of women" is a highly contentious enterprise. This is due in part to the diversity of quite general theoretical perspectives in feminism, all offering different accounts of women's experiences, and in part to the fact that these perspectives have been allied with other theoretical frameworks, such as liberalism, communitarianism, Marxism, or postmodernism. The alliances raise the question of whether there is anything of distinct integrity that emerges from the variety of feminist theories. The answer is best given by setting the question within feminism's recent historical context. By grossly oversimplifying, we can identify what might be called three interactive phases of feminist theory in the United States since about 1970.

Liberal feminism

This approach was most popular during the early phase of the present wave of feminist praxis, but it remains a powerful voice in the ongoing dialogue. Liberal feminism is marked both by its insistence on political, social, and economic equality with men, and by its image of women as mere men who happen to menstruate, gestate, and lactate—biological functions that are held to be morally irrelevant to women's rightful place in society. Consciousness raising allowed women to see that they were being harmed and wronged by patriarchal social structures, but it was liberal conceptions of justice, typically articulated first by men, that helped transform these perceptions into arguments which in turn fueled the struggle for equal rights in the 1970s.[4]

Cultural feminism

By the early 1980s other versions of feminist theory began to challenge the liberal variant; cultural feminism, in particular, is typically regarded as a distinct alternative to liberal feminism and hence may look like a markedly different way of thinking about the world. While liberal feminism affirmed women's likeness to men, cultural feminism stood this presumption on its head, celebrating women's difference from men. Inspired by Carol Gilligan's work on the difference in moral development between men and women, it views women as carers and nurturers whose basic experience of the world importantly includes relationships to vulnerable others.[5] The image of woman underlying the "ethics of care" that emerges here is that of a mother with a baby at her breast—although it is not only the baby but the woman herself who is to be seen as an appropriate object of care.[6] Cultural feminism's powerful insistence on the ethical centrality of women's experience suggests that it must stand out sharply against the backdrop of theorizing dominated by men.[7] But even this strand of feminist thought has strong affinities to standing moral traditions. Its rejection of the Enlightenment view of persons as individualistic, atomic, rational self-interest maximizers and its focus on special, parochial relationships rather than on impartialist, universalizable norms are reminiscent of communitarian and romantic political sensibilities.[8]

Pluralist feminism

Feminism, in both theory and practice, has always tended to be sensitive to differences—paradigmatically, the differences between women and men. Following out this impulse, feminists have recently been focussing more and more attention on differences among women themselves. Both liberal feminism and cultural feminism might ask of a given social policy (such as tying the use of long-term contraceptives to welfare payments), "How does this policy affect women?" In the third phase of recent feminism, which can loosely be termed pluralist feminism, the response would be, "Which women?" The cultural feminists' image of woman as a lactating mother with her baby at her breast was challenged almost as soon as it was advanced,[9] and this challenge picked up considerable theoretical steam later in the 1980s. Cultural feminism in particular was faulted for positing an "essence" of women that transcended class and culture.[10] Women, from a pluralist perspective, are fundamentally different not only from men but also from one another.[11] If we ignore the fact that women are never only women, but also rulers or slaves, artisans or academics, Latinas, African-Americans, or Jews, inhabitants of particular societies in particular eras, then the way feminists use "woman" will be similar to the way in which nonfeminists have used "man": although the stated agenda is to include everybody, one ends by talking only about the needs, interests, and experiences of the dominant, white, middle class. In that contemporary feminist theorists are deeply and creatively engaged with issues of difference, this strand of feminism has clear affinities with other postmodern initiatives to decenter political discourse.

Puzzles of Affinity, Puzzles of Difference

Theorizing feminists have offered many other accounts of what it is to take women's experiences seriously than those canvassed above. But these will do to illustrate the general problems presented by affinities and differences. All feminisms—liberal, cultural, Marxist, pluralist, postmodern, lesbian separatist, dominance, and so on—face the puzzle presented by their affinity to other, nonfeminist bodies of moral theory, and all feminisms face the puzzle of taking note of difference—minimally, noting the difference between women and men. Once difference becomes a category of analysis, it's hard to know when to stop. Even if we realize, for example, that the experiences of homosexual women differ importantly from the experiences of heterosexual women, isn't the inevitable next step to consider whether these particularized categories themselves obscure important differences, say, between older lesbians of color and younger white lesbians? Nor would there seem to be any principled reason why our spade is turned even here. *Any* category seems prone to dissolution: younger white lesbians, for instance, will also be divided by class, religion, and personal experiences. Ultimately, even the integrity of the individual subject—herself "precarious, conflicted, and complex"[12]—is open to theoretical question. The puzzle, then, is to acknowledge the significance of differences among women, while at the same time showing not only that there is some integrity to the concept of "woman," but to feminist theory itself.

Successfully resolving this problem is important for feminism. If there is no core understanding of "woman," then have we any alternative but to return to the atomic individualism with which liberal feminism began?[13] Does the idea of gender-linked injustice—that is, sexism—make sense if there is nothing that women as women have in common by virtue of which they suffer injustice? And if attention to difference dictates that we think in terms of the social classes, families, religions, and ethnic groups in which women are embedded, mightn't we end up valorizing the very communities that have traditionally been the most misogynistic?[14]

The problem of difference in some version or the other seems to trouble all of feminism's varieties. The difference between feminist and nonfeminist thought, then, is merely one variation on this theme—although it is a crucial one. It is crucial because if there is nothing that distinguishes feminist theorizing from other kinds of thought, then it would seem we can do very nicely without feminist theory at all. For those who are skeptical about feminism, this suspicion has raised the issue of whether feminist theories are at best epicycles of theories developed primarily by men—and (except for John Stuart Mill) by men without feminist convictions, at that.[15] If feminist thinking is parasitic on male-generated political, ethical, and social theories, and if there is nothing truly distinctive about feminist thought that puts women at the center of things, then perhaps they weren't so far from the center to begin with.

The flip side of this worry about the difference between feminist thought and the nonfeminist variety is the fear that feminism might be irredeemably tainted by its affinities with male-centered theorizing. Social philosophy, jurisprudence, literary criticism, and the rest are suspected of a thoroughgoing phallocentrism that cannot serve women well. How can Marxist feminism, for example, escape the epistemic and ethical flaws of patriarchy? Psychoanalytic feminism seems to run into the same kind of distinctiveness problem given its reliance on work by Freud, Lacan, and other thinkers who are just as male as Mill, if not more so.[16]

It would seem, then, that even a more adequate presentation than we have provided here of the theoretical riches feminism has to offer is stuck with these two problems:

1. Is there anything at the level of basic theoretical or methodological commitment that distinguishes liberal feminism from liberalism, cultural feminism from communitarianism, pluralist feminism from poststructuralism, and so forth? Isn't it simply a question of adding women to these "isms" and stirring?

2. Is there anything left to feminism at all when one of its most distinctive theoretical impulses—the recognition of difference—is pushed to what seems its logical conclusion—i.e., the elimination of the category of "woman" as a useful theoretical or practical notion? And will this problem not undermine in particular what are ostensibly the most distinctive versions of feminism—dominance views of the kind associated with the work of Catherine McKinnon, which insist that a central, fundamental feature of women's reality is subjugation by men,[17] and radical lesbian separatist feminisms, with their stress on the notion of being "woman-identified"?

These are decidedly living problems in feminist thought. However, we think that a promising way in which all varieties of feminist theory can be distinguished from other "isms" on the one hand, and from disintegrating in the solvent of their own shared sensitivity to difference on the other, is by their traditional commitment to taking women's lived experience seriously as a ground of theorizing. Attention to women's experience can contribute substantially to the soundness of consequentialist moral analysis—to take one example, by illuminating previously obscured consequences of actions and policies and thus permitting a better view of the range of ways in which women have been harmed. Conversely, attending to women's lived experience can thrust into the foreground hitherto unnoticed implications of general deontological frameworks that permit us to see, for example, new respects in which social practices express contempt for women. Attention to women's experience can also reveal the inadequacy of certain images of human agency and interaction that inform a variety of broad ethical theories, thereby permitting challenges to certain ideas that inhere in those theories—for example, the idea that impartiality is a constitutive mark of the moral.[18]

What these remarks amount to is a claim that the proof of feminism is in the pudding: if the importance of feminism as critique is rooted in its ability to challenge the forces that cause clear harms to women, the significance of feminist theory will be expressed in the extent to which it uncovers previously subtle or obscure ways in which women have been ignored and dismissed, and works out the implications of avoiding those subtle harms. The pudding is cooked by means of a feminist commitment related to its insistence on the importance of women's experience: a commitment to the significance of discourse.

Feminist Discourse

The women's movement of the last quarter-century has been marked from the beginning by a careful attention to the ways in which women talk together. This has often involved the telling of stories. The consciousness-raising of the 1970s, for example, took place in groups of women who came together to swap stories about their lives; in the process, a sense of the many ways—some widely shared, some idiosyncratic—in which they had been disadvantaged as women emerged and stood as a basis for both action and reflection. Of all the varieties we have canvassed, much feminist theory recapitulates this practical discipline by its interest in and concern about the forms of conversation available both within communities of feminists and between such communities and the larger society. The dialogic presentation of María Lugones and Elizabeth Spelman's "Have We Got a Theory for You," Carol Gilligan's attention to "voice," Alison Jaggar's current work on the kinds of dialogue employed by feminist activists seeking to change public policy, Ann Ferguson's work in progress on discourses of disagreement, Lorraine Code's *What Can She Know? Feminist Theory and the Construction of Knowledge*—these are only a very random sampling of the attention that feminists have given to discourse. Reflecting on how we talk to one another can help with both the problem of sufficiently individuating feminism from other theories and the problem of too complete a disintegration of the concept of "woman." If feminist theory has been developed in response to and in relationship with what seem tolerably familiar forms of argument, there is nothing so very conventional about the metamorphoses these familiar forms of argument undergo as feminists talk to one another. The discourse itself is often transformative: the arguments, borrowed from other traditions, undergo an alteration in form that changes the nature of the intellectual work feminists are capable of doing.

Traditional forms of argument are altered when they are recast as discourses of coalition-building—or discourses of emotional work,[19] for example—but it's particularly instructive to reflect on what becomes possible for feminist theory when they are recast as narratives. Narrative argumentation permits ethical work to be done up close, so that it engages the emotions and sensibilities. And because it is particularistic, it permits the acknowledgment of rather specific temporal, spatial, and cultural contexts. Working up close changes the nature of the questions that may be asked and offers new strategies for answering them. And when recognition of difference is pushed to its logical conclusion and not only "woman" but "self" dissolves into thin air, narrative can supply the content of women's lived experience that keeps "woman" and "self" from vacuousness—from being neither here nor there.

As a response to the problem of difference, then, feminist narrative proves to be a particularly effective form of discourse. Salient differences and differences within differences are allowed to emerge from story telling and story listening—that is, they come out of experiences as opposed to being imposed on experience by theory. Salient commonalities emerge; the women in the consciousness-raising group, or those who form the audience for the article, hear the stories speak to and illuminate aspects of their own lives. Valuable dispositions attendant on the proper use of narrative—empathy and imagination—are reinforced, thus further helping us resist both premature moves toward commonality and excessive skepticism about what is shared.[20]

Feminist discourses of all kinds become a device for allowing difference its protean but not imperialist scope. They do so not least by reminding us that there are frameworks within which all conversations go on. The framework that feminism insists on is still quite viable after we attend carefully to the differences in women's lives: what emerges from these shared stories is an overlapping consensus that—in a multitude of ways—women are treated unfairly, disrespectfully, and harmfully by virtue of their being women, that this state of affairs is wrong, and that it must end. It cannot end until we are clearer about the many ways in which unjust treatment expresses itself in the lives of women whose experiences are also shaped by the other factors that constitute their identity. Attention to this framework is something like G. E. Moore's gesture refuting philosophical skepticism: arguing against skeptics motivated by philosophical idealism, he held up his hands, so demonstrating that at least two physical objects exist in the external world.[21] Concrete experience of commonalities and differences are more trustworthy than the far-flung theoretical dialectics driving the difference view to its extremes, just as Moore's demonstration was more trustworthy than the arguments of the idealists. This, of course, does not mean that there is no place for probing skepticism or fine-grained sensitivity to difference. Rather, the moral is that such proclivities be put in the service of productive thinking about real problems rather than be permitted to derail such thinking.

In what follows, we will show how attention to discourse supports the fashioning of a tool for shedding new light on the ethics of certain public policy employments of long-term contraceptives.

A Feminist-Theoretic Tool for Assessing Contraceptive Policy

A concern for *women's* lived experience and a belief that the unjust marginalization and oppression of women shapes our lives in very fundamental ways prompts the question: how does the use of long-term contraceptives affect our understanding of women's role in procreation, in rearing children, and in other aspects of social life? The question orients us to attend to the meanings of being a woman in a society that is laid out with the convenience of middle- and upper-class men in mind and to how long-term contraceptives might alter those patterns of meaning.

Like many societies, our own has forged iron links between women's procreative capacity, the nurturing of children, and limitations on other forms of social expression and reward. Here as elsewhere, being female has implied bearing children; being female and bearing children has typically implied almost full responsibility for the children's upbringing; being female, bearing children, and having near-total responsibility for their upbringing has excluded women from full participation in business, the arts, higher education, the professions, and other forms of social expression, activity, and reward. To a significant degree, this exclusion takes place whether or not the woman has in fact borne children. We regard the links between reproductive capacity, unjust apportioning of responsibilites for rearing, and consequent social exclusion as part of the common framework in which the individual narratives of many women's lives are played out; they are part of what is meant when we say that women as women have been harmed, wronged, or treated unfairly.

Aggregating childbearing with a seriously disproportionate amount of responsibility for child rearing has contributed to women's oppression. Corporate life, for example, is still largely structured on the premise that the executive as well as the assembly-line worker has a wife at home who is taking care of the kids. And among the very poor, where staying home with the kids has never been an option, women are nevertheless expected to provide whatever care is available, even if this means they must forgo certain opportunities such as schooling to improve the quality of their lives. Men are not expected to do the same. The links between childbearing (but not inseminating) and social roles are built directly into the way female children are socialized. They have a profound influence on the answers available when women ask Kant's durable trinity of questions: What can I know? What should I do? And what may I hope for?

In saying this, we don't mean to argue that givers of birth are not or should not be mothers—namely, nurturers and protectors of their young. But inseminators as well as childbearers have a responsibility to nurture their offspring. As Sara Ruddick has argued, this is properly called maternal work, and men are equally obliged to do it.[22] Yet men do not fulfill this obligation in anything like an equal share with women. Indeed, for men the link between the capacity to procreate and the obligation to rear is so weak that it not infrequently snaps altogether.[23] A feminist ethics, starting from women's experience, will note that just as the connection between childbearing and nurturing has been systematically exaggerated and so kept all women, not only mothers, from full participation in the public sphere, so by contrast the connection between siring a child and nurturing it has been systematically underplayed to the detriment of children and women alike. In a world where men and women both are parents, the social arrangements produced by this difference in meaning between men's and women's procreative capacities are morally inadequate.

Now, by situating women's power to procreate within this social context that gives it meaning and asking whether that meaning has contributed to women's well-being, we have manufactured a feminist tool suitable to the analysis of the social policy uses of long-acting contraceptives: the tool is to note where childbearing is unfairly aggregated with bearing the brunt of child-rearing responsibilities to the exclusion of other social opportunities and to disaggregate these responsibilities wherever possible.

Reproductive Disaggregation and Liberal Theory: Norplant as a Condition of Probation

How is "reproductive disaggregation" a distinctively feminist tool? Mightn't other political theories have come up with the same strategy? This is, of course, possible. But the distinctiveness of feminist theory does not depend upon the logical uniqueness of its results. As a matter of fact, because they are not focusing on women per se, other critical perspectives are apt to miss just precisely the aggregation of procreative ability in women, but not in men, with certain social roles that our analysis has noted. We want to show how this can happen by putting our tool to work on two concerns regarding social policies involving long-acting contraception and comparing our results with those arrived at when one applies other theoretical tools that are also ready to hand.

The first concern we want to take up is the rightfulness of using Norplant as a condition of probation. This question can be tackled with a pretty straightforwardly liberal set of tools—liberal in that they shape the question in terms of social constraint and individual freedoms as these notions are understood to affect people in general. The argument, which is considered in the work of John Robertson,[24] goes like this:

1. A person who commits child abuse may justly be sentenced to a term in prison.
2. While in prison, the child abuser is deprived of many liberties, including the liberty to procreate.
3. Since being deprived of the liberty to procreate is a lesser punishment than being in prison, and the greater punishment includes the lesser, it is therefore just to deprive a child abuser of her liberty to procreate while she is on probation rather than in prison.

It is worth noting that the position defended here is actually stronger than required to address the incidents that have in fact occurred. A woman convicted of child abuse was offered the use of Norplant as a condition of parole; if she had chosen against having the contraceptive implanted, then she had the alternative of jail.[25] If the argument "whatever justifies coercive removal of liberty also justifies coercive removal of the ability to procreate" goes through, then offering women the *option* of using Norplant (rather than coercing them into using it) may seem very strongly justified indeed. But consider the following argument, which relies on the reproductive-rearing disaggregation strategy:

1. A person who commits child abuse can justly be sentenced to a term in prison.
2. While in prison, the child abuser is deprived of many liberties, including the liberty to procreate.
3. Being deprived of the liberty to procreate may be a lesser punishment than being in prison, but to punish child abuse directly through this deprivation (rather than having the loss of procreative opportunities be one of a range of limits to liberty, foreseen, but not, as it were, intended) has the expressive function of reinforcing the unfair aggregation of the childbearing and child-rearing functions. The point of the contraception in this case is not to keep women from *having* children; it is to keep them from *abusing* children. That is an off-label use of Norplant. It is not her reproductive capability that the woman wielded badly, but her power to act as a safe primary caregiver for her children. These are two distinct capabilities that, given common and destructive themes in the social construction of femininities, need to be clearly

seen and acknowledged as distinct. So making Norplant a condition of probation is not justified. A judge would do better to rule that an abusive mother must work a demanding job outside the home while the child's father attends to the primary child care responsibilities.

Now, we aren't claiming that this conclusion necessarily trumps the other; we're merely demonstrating that it's different. And we are pointing out that nonfeminist liberal theory is likely to miss the unfair aggregation feature of the problem.

What would be involved in showing that the disaggregation concern was morally more significant than the "greater includes the lesser" approach? One strategy would be to try to compare consequences: would the harm caused to women by reinforcing the unfair aggregation of childbearing and child rearing outweigh whatever good would be done by offering convicted female child abusers Norplant as a condition of probation? Like most consequentialist approaches to morally difficult questions, the answer to this is not easy to see. However, another strategy is to cast the question deontologically: is the aggregation of childbearing and child rearing not only a structure that harms women, but also one that insults them? Is suggesting that a woman's procreative role is to be regarded as far more closely involved with child rearing than a man's itself a serious expression of disrespect, not merely to the woman who stands before the judge, but to women in general?

We believe the Norplant offer is both harmful and disrespectful to women generally; in order to justify offering long-term contraception as a condition of probation, it would have to be clear that the benefits to be obtained by doing so were extremely significant and unlikely to be obtained by other, less harmful or disrespectful methods (such as providing the woman with demanding work outside the home while the child care is provided by the father). It would not be enough simply to point to the "lesser is included in the greater" argument; sometimes, less *is* more. If this is right, then a feminist analysis points out morally relevant differences that a nonfeminist liberal approach fails to note.

Reproductive Disaggregation and Communitarian Theory: Norplant in the Schools

CURE, a clergy group in East Baltimore speaking on behalf of the African-American community, has raised serious reservations concerning the use of Norplant for teenagers. A broadside they distributed offers a number of arguments against the contraceptive, not the least forceful of which is an argument whose theoretical basis is a kind of separatism: the African-American community has suffered so much oppression at the hands of the dominant white culture that it is surely right to be deeply suspicious of that culture's solutions to the problem of black teenage pregnancy.

But we want to focus on another argument we find in the broadside— an argument with communitarian underpinnings. It goes like this:

1. Culture in the black community . . . sees the birth of a baby as a joyous occasion. Many young people choose to have babies and most take care of them quite well.
2. The majority culture may not understand our community's values.
3. Therefore the majority culture ought to leave the management of procreation within our community to the community itself, so that the community's culture and family values are promoted.[26]

Here again the application of our feminist tool yields a different conclusion:

1. Culture in the black community sees the birth of a baby as a joyous occasion. Many young *girls* choose to have babies and most take care of them quite well, with the help of their *mothers and grandmothers*.
2. The black *community's* dominant interpreters—the male clergy—may not understand the *individual narratives* that make up the lives of these women.
3. To assume that the young girls in the black community, as in the majority culture, have primary responsibility for rearing the babies they bear is to aggregate childbearing with primary child rearing. Because this aggregation perpetuates social structures that favor men at women's expense, neither the majority culture *nor* the black community are in a position to manage procreation so that it does not oppress the community's teenage girls. The clergy may be interpreting many of the community's values correctly, but the teenage girls, their mothers, and their grandmothers may have other interests that are not well served by that interpretation.

A pluralist feminist might wonder whether we aren't illicitly smuggling in the interests of white middle-class women when we suggest that aggregating childbearing, caring for children, and limited access with other social functions runs counter to women's interests. But she would have a similar concern about the appeal to *the* values of the black community: are the interests of black women well represented in that appeal? Sorting out this issue would be a difficult task, but if the claim that the oppression of women is endemic in all cultures is true—and the evidence seems overwhelming— then embedding the management of female reproductive activities even further into a given community is, on the face of it, not likely to forward women's interests.

Note that the conclusion here differs from the conclusion respecting Norplant as a condition of probation. In the case of probation, the judge's offer carries the expressive force that women's responsibilities to their offspring are different from men's. In the case of the Baltimore community, the clergy's attack suggests that they falsely totalize the experience of African-Americans. In trying to keep long-term contraception away from young women in their community, the clergy suppose that everyone in that community upholds the social convention that links sexual activity between women and men to a set of responsibilities that must be met, and that everyone is content with the system of assigning to mothers and other women the brunt of these responsibilities. But if this unjust social arrangement is in fact affirmed only by those it serves best, then Norplant might be just what is required to defend girls and women of the community against it. The contraceptive can protect young girls in particular from some of the damaging social consequences of the sex-gender system in which they live.

A Question of Choice: Dollar-a-Day Programs and Family Matters

This pattern of analysis may suggest that a feminist perspective on long-term contraception is fundamentally voluntarist: if women want to use Norplant, this ought to be allowed and expedited, since it gives them power against the special burdens society attaches to women's sexuality, while coercively inducing them to accept the contraceptive expresses an endorsement of those special burdens, which is a reason to suppose we ought not to engage in policies of coercion.

We want to close by considering two further cases that will complicate this voluntaristic picture. One concerns the extent to which social programs may use milder incentives for encouraging women to use long-acting contraceptives; the other focuses on the possibility that interests other than those of the women in question might be appropriate grounds for inducements for using some such devices.

In 1985 Planned Parenthood of the Rocky Mountains, the Denver Children's Home, and the Denver Children's Hospital pioneered "Dollar-a-Day," a program to provide teenage girls who already had one child with a mild incentive to avoid a second pregnancy. Five years later, the program's scope was expanded to help girls at high risk for a primary pregnancy as well. By 1992 there were five such groups of approximately fifteen girls each. The groups, led by trained adolescent counsellors, meet once a week at a neighborhood health station to offer moral support, promote self-esteem, and broaden the girls' visions of what their futures can be. A girl receives seven dollars weekly for participating in the two-year program, but her membership is terminated if she becomes pregnant. Do these programs contribute to or dismantle the social link between bearing and rearing that can be so damaging to females?

Let's press this question by considering the contraceptive that is used. Instead of condoms, birth control pills, diaphragms, or abstinence, let's suppose the girl uses a long-term contraceptive. In a manner of speaking, of course, Dollar-a-Day programs are themselves a form of long-term contraception in that the goal is to avoid pregnancy for two years. The difference between these programs and, say, Norplant, is that social, rather than biomedical, means are used to achieve the long-term goal. But suppose a passive, biomedical long-term contraceptive were used in addition to the Dollar-a-Day incentive. Suppose, instead of $7 a week, these same teenage girls were offered $100 four times a year for accepting a shot of Depo-Provera. Because this agent is active for three months per injection, the incentive is still roughly a dollar a day, but the sum is now large enough to represent a fairly powerful inducement. To repeat the question, would a Dollar-a-Day Depo-Provera program aggregate or disaggregate the link between childbearing and child rearing?

It seems to us that a program of this sort could be seen much as we have presented the Baltimore program: as trying to defend young women against some of the damaging consequences of the sex-gender framework in which they live, while still providing them with some deliberative space in which to reflect on the appropriateness of Depo-Provera in their own particular narrative. However, it would be much preferable if the program in question didn't merely acquiesce in the present construction of parental responsibility for rearing children, but also tried to attack it. Why shouldn't a Dollar-a-Day program for avoiding pregnancy among girls be complemented by mild-incentive programs targeted to boys? These could be designed both to increase boys' sexual responsibility and to encourage teenage fathers to accept *their* fair share of responsibility. If mild inducements to use long-acting contraceptives were combined with other activities that explicitly try to discourage not just pregnancy, but the bad social consequences of pregnancy for very young women, they would be immensely more palatable. A feminist analysis highlights the importance of placing social policy uses of long-acting contraceptives within an appropriate context: one in which boys are induced to take responsibility for their sexuality as well. Contextualizing the question of inducements for accepting Depo-Provera makes it easier to see that taking care not to coerce girls to avoid pregnancy is not the only moral consideration at issue here.

If society has a legitimate role in defending girls against the untoward effects of unjust distributions of parental responsibility by encouraging both girls and boys to avoid conception and by encouraging boys to accept some of the burdens of parenthood should they become fathers, what role should families play here? Since this is a very large question, let's focus on a situation that features some particularly interesting problems for family authority in this respect.

Imagine a young girl, Amy, who at age thirteen is raped by an acquaintance and, as a result, conceives. She is adamant that abortion is out of the question; she has "already bonded" with "her baby." What is more, as her parents explore her options with her, it becomes clear that the rape was not her first sexual experience, and they come to think there is little they can do to discourage her from having a very heterosexually active adolescence.

Happily, Amy soon has a miscarriage. She is not in principle opposed to contraception, but she sometimes speaks longingly of "her lost child," and her mother, Sara, is very frightened that she may forget to take her birth control pills or to insist that her partners use condoms. Sara suggests to Amy that she use a long-acting contraceptive in addition to condoms, but Amy thinks the idea of Norplant is gross and even objects to having an injection of Depo-Provera four times a year—she hates shots. Do her parents have any moral standing to insist that Amy have the injection every three months?

An argument in favor of such a position can stem from the feminist disaggregation standpoint. While it might seem odd to justify what could amount to a coercive use of contraceptives on feminist grounds, a little attention to the differences among women quickly reveals that when very young teenagers are pregnant, the burden of rearing the children of these children is typically carried by older women—their mothers and other female relatives. This would surely be the case for Amy and Sara, since Amy is more irresponsible than even the average thirteen-year-old, and Amy's father has a demanding job that involves a great deal of travel.

While an alternative to forced contraception might be to allow Amy's parents to insist that any of Amy's children be placed for adoption, the costs to Amy—and perhaps to her children as well—of exerting such authority involve, if anything, even more coercion than the insistence on getting one shot every three months and putting up with the ensuing changes in periodicity.

It seems to us reasonable to believe that Amy's parents do have the moral standing to insist that their daughter undergo a very mild invasion of her body to protect both Amy and Sara against major negative consequences in their lives. They might begin by pointing out to Amy that the brunt of the child care would fall on Sara. They might appeal to Amy's sense of fairness and to her sense of how uncool it is to be saddled with a kid in junior high. They might point out that if there's a baby, that means less money and time to spend on Amy. They might bribe, threaten, or ground Amy; manipulate her; or try to figure out what is missing from her life that makes the idea of a baby so attractive. What they certainly will *not* do is couch the question along standard liberal lines, seeing it as a matter of Amy's uncoerced reproductive choice. As a safeguard against abuse of parental authority, we would propose that some form of social scrutiny—a court review, perhaps—be put in place in these cases. Where long-acting contraception is requested for a girl over her objections, the court could be asked to determine that there is in fact good reason to believe that she is heterosexually active, that she will not reliably use contraceptives in her own behalf, that the burden of rearing her children would fall disproportionately on others, and that the use of the contraceptive will not put her at any appreciable risk.

Coda: Some Concluding Practical and Theoretical Considerations

We reiterate that the disaggregation perspective we have offered as a distinctly feminist approach to questions of social uses of long-acting contraceptives is meant only to place a morally significant element of the problem into the arena of ethical deliberation, not to resolve the issue; other concerns are relevant as well. However, those other concerns—for example, how we analyze the difference between encouragement, inducement, and coercion; whether health care professionals are appropriate agents of social policy; and what reasons we have to trust social power as it is brought to bear on women given society's less than shining record in this regard—are all also fields for feminist scrutiny and theorizing.

This theorizing doesn't go on in a vacuum; it is both supported by and constrained within the social context in which it occurs. In fact, as we have argued, it shapes and is shaped by the discourse that goes on in that context. But it is crucial that we not confound it *with* that context—that we resist the temptation to subsume feminism too quickly under the other modes of theorizing that are practiced in its societal context. If we misunderstand the ability of feminist theory to make a distinctive contribution to the debate over the social uses of long-term contraception, we will have an important set of resources for making wise decisions in this area directly under our noses— but we won't think to use them.

NOTES

1. A clear and oft-quoted statement of feminism's fundamental insight is that of Alison Jaggar, "Feminist Ethics: Problems, Projects, Prospects," in *Feminist Ethics*, ed. Claudia Card (Lawrence: University Press of Kansas, 1991), 95. For a thoughtful analysis of how such oppression is wrong, see Iris Marion Young's *Justice and the Politics of Difference* (Princeton: Princeton University Press, 1990), especially 53–54.

2. See John A. Robertson, "Norplant and Irresponsible Reproduction," this volume, 79–107.

3. For an excellent discussion of this exclusion and how it occurred, see Genevieve Lloyd, *The Man of Reason: "Male" and "Female" in Western Philosophy* (Minneapolis: University of Minnesota Press, 1984).

4. A good academic work in this genre is Janet Radcliffe Richards's *The Sceptical Feminist* (Harmondsworth, U.K.: Penguin, 1980).

5. In addition to her classic *In a Different Voice* (Cambridge, Mass.: Harvard University Press, 1982), see also Carol Gilligan, "Moral Orientation and Moral Development," in *Women and Moral Theory*, ed. Eva Feder Kittay and Diana T. Meyers (Totowa, N.J.: Rowman and Littlefield, 1987), 19–36.

6. An admirable exemplar of the ethics of care is Sara Ruddick, *Maternal Thinking: Toward a Politics of Peace* (Boston: Beacon Press, 1989).

7. See Nel Noddings, *Caring* (Berkeley and Los Angeles: University of California Press, 1984) and the critique by Hilde Lindemann Nelson, "Against Caring," *Journal of Clinical Ethics* 3, no. 1 (1992): 8–15.

8. An excellent criticism of the Enlightenment view of persons is Virginia Held's "Non-Contractual Society," in *Science, Morality, and Feminist Theory*, ed. Marsha Hanen and Kai Nielsen, supplementary volume 13 of the *Canadian Journal of Philosophy* (Calgary: University of Calgary Press, 1987).

9. Bernice Johnson Reagon, for example, argued that "the women's movement has perpetuated a myth that there is some common experience that comes just cause you're women." See "Coalition Politics: Turning the Century," in *Home Girls: A Black Feminist Anthology*, ed. Barbara Smith (New York: Kitchen Table/Women of Color Press, 1983), 360.

10. A scathing critique of essentialism was mounted by María C. Lugones and Elizabeth V. Spelman in "Have We Got a Theory for You! Feminist Theory, Cultural Imperialism, and the Demand for 'The Woman's Voice,'" in *Women's Studies International Forum* 6, no. 6 (1983): 573–81. This was followed by Spelman's *Inessential Woman: Problems of Exclusion in Feminist Thought* (Boston: Beacon Press, 1988).

11. See Denise Riley, *"Am I That Name?" Feminism and the Category of "Women" in History* (Minneapolis: University of Minnesota Press, 1988).

12. Patricia Elliot, *From Mastery to Analysis: Theories of Gender in Psychoanalytic Feminism* (Ithaca, N.Y.: Cornell University Press, 1991), 75.

13. This possibility is discussed by Anne C. Dailey, "Feminism's Return to Liberalism," *Yale Law Review* 102 (1993): 1265–86.

14. See Marilyn Friedman's "Feminism and Modern Friendship: Dislocating the Community," *Ethics* 99 (January 1989): 275–90.

15. Although Mill is the great exception to the claim about significant male theorists lacking feminist sympathies, Annette Baier has tried to make a case for David Hume, too; see her "Hume, The Women's Moral Theorist?" in Kittay and Meyers, 37–55.

16. For an example of feminist misgivings directed against feminist borrowings from psychoanalysis, see Judith Antrobut's review essay, "In the Final Analysis," *Women's Review of Books* 4 (February 1987).

17. See Catherine McKinnon, *Feminism Unmodified* (Cambridge, Mass.: Harvard University Press, 1987); but see also Angela P. Harris, "Race and Essentialism in Feminist Legal Theory," *Stanford Law Review* 42 (1990): 581–616.

18. For a very nice discussion of this point, see Annette Baier, "What Do Women Want in a Moral Theory?" *Nous* 19 (March 1985); Held's "Non-Contractual Society" mounts the challenge directly as well.

19. Reagon, "Coalition Politics"; Cheshire Calhoun, "Emotional Work," in *Explorations in Feminist Ethics*, ed. Eve Browning Cole and Susan Coultrap-McQuin (Bloomington: Indiana University Press, 1992), 117–22.

20. For further discussion and application of narrative as a response to the problem of difference, see Hilde Lindemann Nelson, "Resistance and Insubordination," *Hypatia* 10, no. 2 (Spring 1995): 23–40. See also Dailey, "Feminism's Return to Liberalism."

21. G. E. Moore, "A Proof of the External World," *Proceedings of the British Academy* 25 (1939), reprinted in Moore's *Philosophical Papers* (London: George Allen and Unwin, 1959).

22. Ruddick, *Maternal Thinking*, 42–45.

23. For the depressing statistics supporting this claim see, among others, Susan Moller Okin, *Justice, Gender, and the Family* (New York: Basic Books, 1989), especially chapter 7. A recent study conducted at the University of Pennsylvania reported that half the children surveyed five years after divorce had not heard from their fathers for at least a year. The *New York Times* account of the study (31 August 1993) entitled, "More and More, the Single Parent Is Dad," noted that fathers now head 14% of single-parent households, up from 10% in 1980. It follows that 86% of single-parent households are headed by women.

24. John Robertson, *Children of Choice: Freedom and the New Reproductive Technologies* (Princeton: Princeton University Press, 1994), 82–83.

25. A week after Norplant received FDA approval for use in the United States, Darlene Johnson was ordered to accept it as a condition of probation after being convicted of child abuse. The case is described in detail by Stacey Arthur, "The Norplant Prescription: Birth control, Woman Control, or Crime Control?" *UCLA Law Review* 40 (1992): 1–101, 15–19.

26. CURE, "Information on and Concerns about Norplant in the Black Community," undated but circulated about 15 January 1993, photocopy.

PART IV: International Perspectives

RUTH MACKLIN
Cultural Difference and Long-Acting Contraception

TOLA OLU PEARCE
Ethical Issues in the Importation of Long-Acting Contraceptives to Nigeria

ELLEN HARDY
Long-Acting Contraception in Brazil and the Dominican Republic

RUTH MACKLIN

Cultural Difference and Long-Acting Contraception

Cultural values influence the choices individuals make in many areas of their lives. Yet it is important not to overestimate the influence of cultural values compared to other factors that shape individual behavior, especially in the area of human reproduction. In support of this position, I propose two main theses:

1. Although a woman's use of contraceptives may be influenced by cultural values, her behavior regarding contraceptives is actually determined by a combination of government policies, the practices of individual health care providers with whom she comes in contact, and the degree to which she has freedom from control by her sexual partner(s); and
2. In developed as well as developing countries, the social and economic class to which a woman belongs, rather than cultural values, is what shapes the extent to which government policies and providers' actions affect a particular woman's use of contraceptives.

Many diverse factors contribute to how individuals behave with regard to controlling their reproductive lives and their use of contraceptives. On the African continent, for example, men have typically rejected condoms even if they are prepared to accept the use of contraceptives by their wives. In contrast, condom use is very high among Japanese men; condoms are the favorite method of contraception among Japanese couples.[1] To cite a different example, the high abortion rates in the former Soviet-bloc countries of Eastern Europe are explained not by a cultural value embracing abortion, but rather by a very low rate of contraceptive use. The reason for that, in turn, is not a cultural value rejecting contraceptives but simply their unavailability to the population during the years of socialist rule.

The worldwide prevalence of abortion is another illustration of the point. Cultural values in many countries oppose or prohibit abortion, yet women in every stratum of every society, including practicing Roman Catholics, seek and undergo abortions in order to terminate unwanted pregnancies. It is evident that the individual desire of millions of women not to be pregnant overrides their religious or cultural value that deplores abortion.

Benefits and Risks of Long-term Methods

The wide array of contraceptives now approved for use in both developing and developed countries can be hailed as a triumph of medical science, making possible unprecedented control of fertility. This impressive array is also a potential boon for freedom of choice, enabling individuals to choose a method of family planning that accords with their personal or cultural values. Long-acting methods of contraception afford users the opportunity to undergo a one-time procedure that regulates fertility for weeks, months, or years.

Yet the very same factors that confer benefits on individuals can also lead to their being harmed or wronged. The introduction of long-term contraception frees the user from the need to ingest a daily pill or deal with barrier methods at the time of sexual relations. Yet it also opens the door to control over individuals' choices by governments, family-planning programs, or health care providers. Whether in the form of a nonhormonal device (standard IUD), a hormonal method (Depo-Provera or Norplant), or a combination (hormone-releasing IUD), long-acting contraceptives can result in limitations on control by the user.

The wide range of contraceptives now available is accompanied by an equally wide array of individual and cultural values and attitudes toward their use. Some values affecting contraceptive choice can be traced directly to the culture or subculture in which they are traditionally embedded, while others are superimposed from without. An example of the former is the rejection by women from some cultural and religious groups of methods that cause irregular bleeding throughout the menstrual cycle. Their reason for rejecting these methods stems, in part, from conformity to a religious or cultural prohibition forbidding sexual intercourse during menstruation.

An example of a transcultural, superimposed value is the rejection of hormonal methods by women's activists in many countries. Following the lead of international feminist groups such as FINRRAGE (Feminist International Network of Resistance to Reproductive and Genetic Engineering),[2] women's health activists in developing countries are strongly opposed to a variety of new reproductive technologies. Their opposition to the introduction of Norplant and Depo-Provera into family planning programs stems not from the fact that these methods are long-acting, but from the circumstance that they work by altering the woman's natural hormonal system. The value that prompts their rejection is "adherence to nature." Hormonal methods interfere with nature in a way that barrier methods of contraception do not.

Although this attack has been mounted primarily against Norplant and Depo-Provera (long-acting methods), opposition has been voiced by these same groups to one-time or as-needed use of RU-486 for fertility regulation. The same arguments presumably apply to oral contraceptives, which are hormonal in their action but nevertheless user controlled.

Values pertaining to the use of contraception may therefore vary according to culture, religion, ideology, and individual preference. What appears to be universal is the desire of women throughout the world to regulate the number and spacing of their children. What varies from circumstance to circumstance and from individual to individual are the factors that influence their use of contraceptives and whether women are afforded a choice among methods.

Ethical and policy considerations will differ according to whether a government has instituted a population control program, whether a variety of contraceptive methods are readily available to users, and whether family planning programs promote some methods over others. From the perspective of individual contraceptive users, it may make a difference whether a method is reversible or irreversible, long-term or short-term, hormonal or nonhormonal, user-controlled versus provider-controlled, woman-controlled as opposed to requiring the cooperation of her partner, and when in a woman's reproductive life it is to be employed.

The ethical and policy considerations posed by long-acting methods are directly related to the opportunity of women to choose freely. When there is complete freedom of choice, and people have ready access to contraceptive information and services, including safe removal of a long-acting method such as an IUD or implant, no special ethical concerns are likely to arise. But when people have little or no choice among alternative contraceptive methods, or if a method can be imposed without an individual's knowledge or consent, then long-term methods have the potential for abuse. That would result in unwarranted intrusion into people's reproductive lives and value preferences.

Two ethically relevant considerations pertain to long-acting contraceptives. The first flows from the well-established requirements of informed consent—namely, that consent must be informed and it must be voluntary. If women are not told that a long-acting, hormonal method is likely to produce irregular bleeding, they have not been adequately informed. If women with multiple sexual partners are not told about their risk of pelvic inflammatory disease and subsequent infertility in the event they contract a sexually transmitted disease, they have not been adequately informed. And obviously, if women are not told that an injection being administered is a contraceptive that lasts for three months, their consent is not voluntary.

The second ethically relevant consideration relates to the prospect for safe, timely removal of a long-acting contraceptive device or implant. Even if a woman's consent to insert or implant a contraceptive is adequately informed and fully voluntary, it is not ethically valid unless the opportunity exists for removal at her discretion. She may seek removal because of the desire to become pregnant sooner than she had anticipated when the device or implant was inserted. Or she may have a change in her life circumstances, such as having entered a new relationship with accompanying uncertainty regarding the transmission of sexually transmitted diseases. Or she may find the side effects of the long-acting method unacceptable. In some developing countries, women have had difficulty finding physicians willing to remove an IUD, and the skill required to remove an implant may be lacking even in physicians who have been properly taught to insert the implant. In this regard, injectables have the advantage of not requiring removal by a skilled and willing provider.

From an ethical point of view, it is important to identify the basis for concerns about newly introduced contraceptives. The concern of women's health advocates opposed to hormonal methods is that women may be harmed by taking exogenous substances that interfere with the natural regulation of the body. The concern of those opposed to long-acting methods is that women may be wronged through lack of informed consent, by being coerced, and by the absence of trained or skilled providers to do a proper removal.

Cultural Values: Why People Have Children

Having children is a significant value in most cultures, even more important in some than in others. It may well be paramount among some ethnic groups or subcultures in the United States as it has been for many centuries in China, Mexico, and among pronatalist religious groups. A philosophy professor from Nigeria has written that "Africans generally place a high value on children. A human life is not considered full without them. It is part of the determinants of personhood. The main purpose of marriage is to have children and increase the honor of the clan."[3]

Cultural values deeply influence the behavior of couples with regard to having children in China, Mexico, and the Philippines.[4] During a visit I made to China, two Chinese philosophers provided a background for understanding the importance people attach to having children, especially sons. A Chinese cultural tradition that goes back 5000 years is the culture-laden notion of "filial piety." This concept dictates respect for parents. It can be traced to Confucius, who said, "Without a son there is a great problem." As one of these Chinese philosophers wrote:

According to traditional Chinese belief, not having a child results from not having virtue. In fact, the most serious violation of the Confucian principle of filial piety is to be without offspring. A Chinese man without a child experiences heavy psychological pressure, and the burden is especially onerous for women because infertility is always blamed on the wife. Wives who do not bear a child are stigmatized and mistreated—even abused—in families that stick to traditional values.[5]

Originating in this ancient tradition, the idea of family lineage is still important. It remains especially strong in rural areas. Furthermore, sons are important for labor in the countryside. One of the philosophers said that historically, manpower has been very important in China; this is the chief reason for controversy over family planning in China. The "one couple, one child" policy has been said to conflict with the government's economic goals in the countryside. These latter goals "put a premium on improved agricultural productivity and thereby make additional children who can help in the fields valuable assets. It also clashes with traditional Chinese culture and with the wishes of peasants."[6]

Information obtained in the Philippines suggests a different set of factors explaining why couples living in overpopulated countries who already have several children continue to have more children. As in Mexico and China, traditional beliefs and practices comprise part of the explanation. In addition, 85% of the population is Roman Catholic, with many devout adherents to official Catholic teachings regarding reproduction.

IUDs are not widely accepted in the Philippines because some people, including many physicians and politicians, consider them an abortifacient. IUDs have also received bad press and distorted reports by the media. The government has not approved implants as part of family planning programs, in part because of a lack of "political will," an attorney explained. It has been an ongoing battle in the Philippines to get family planning accepted. This is largely because of strong opposition by the powerful Catholic church. Recent surveys show, however, that 80% of all Filipinos approve of a campaign to promote the use of artificial contraception launched by Dr. Juan Flavier, the current Philippine health secretary in the administration of Fidel Ramos.[7]

A general problem with the use of contraceptives as described by one Filipino physician is the failure of women to use the methods about which they are informed at the family planning clinic. There is especially poor compliance in using the pill. Some women are afraid of cancer; others seem simply to deny that they will become pregnant: they believe that the rhythm method is an effective means of birth control. An attorney working in the area of reproductive rights provided another explanation: a tendency toward fatalism as a general cultural trait among Filipinos. Many Filipinos believe that "God will take care of things," an attitude reflected in the broader cultural phenomenon of lack of planning for the future. A widespread belief among less-educated Filipinos is that people are generally unable to control their lives. Severe weather phenomena and volcanic eruptions over which they have no control contribute to this tendency toward fatalism. Having many children is no more subject to the control of individuals than is an eruption of Mount Pinatubo.

A special barrier exists in the Philippines for some women who seek sterilization as a way not to have any more children when their desired family size is complete. The barrier is the "spousal consent" ("spousal authorization" is the preferred term) generally required by clinics or health providers as a condition of performing tubal ligations.[8] I asked an attorney from the Institute of Judicial Administration in Manila whether spousal authorization is required by law and if not, whether it is nevertheless widely practiced. The attorney said that the family code does not require consent of a spouse for a partner's sterilization; however, family planning clinics do, as a matter of fact, always require spousal consent. It is sometimes (mistakenly) argued that the law requires spousal authorization, but those who make such arguments are either ignorant of the law or deliberately misrepresenting it.

Requiring spousal authorization for a woman's sterilization reflects a traditional value that enables husbands to control their wives' fertility. That family planning clinics continue to subscribe to this practice, despite the fact that it is not a legal requirement, reveals adherence to the cultural pattern of male dominance and lack of respect for women's autonomy. Thus, despite the preference of the individual woman to undergo an irreversible, long-acting contraceptive method, she is prevented from acting in accordance with her own values by medical practitioners upholding a cultural custom that cannot be defended as a matter of ethical principle.

In Mexico, anecdotal accounts from women activists revealed that the dominant value of "machismo" creates in men the desire to prove their masculinity by having many children. Indeed, whether it is their wives or their mistresses who bear the children, macho credit goes to the men for fathering numerous offspring. In general, Mexican culture places a high value on family and children, yet as is true everywhere, individual women seek to control their fertility.

One Mexican social anthropologist writes that the prevalent values of patriarchal Mexican culture make the roles of motherhood and fatherhood central elements in the gender construction of masculinity and femininity: "Until recent years, popular sayings included: 'To be a man is to be the father of more than four.'"[9] A saying pertaining to women is considerably less charitable: "Women . . . were to be kept 'like shotguns, loaded and in the corner'. That is to say, pregnant and marginalized when it came to important matters."[10] Information provided by social scientists and women's health advocates revealed that in many cases women seek to limit family size while their husbands, with strong support from the husbands' mothers, compel the wives to continue to have children.

Similar power of the woman's mother-in-law came to light in China. One example was provided at a meeting with representatives from the State Family Planning Commission by a medical college graduate who now works as an administrator in the Commission.

A woman in a village had three children, all girls. She did not want more children, but her husband and mother-in-law did not want her to be sterilized. They wanted her to continue having children at least until she had a son. The ethical issue was presented as a dilemma for the physician: should she sterilize the woman? or follow the wishes of the patient's husband and mother-in-law? The physician tried to persuade the mother-in-law and husband to agree to the woman's sterilization, but that attempt failed.

What would be the consequences for the woman if the physician counselled her to go ahead with the sterilization? Everyone at the meeting concurred that the consequence would be that the husband would divorce her. Since the husband and mother-in-law wanted sons in the family, the husband would have to divorce a sterilized wife and get himself a new wife who might bear him sons.

What then would be the consequence to the woman following a divorce? She would be rejected from the family and lose whatever possessions she had—including custody of her own children, who would remain with their father and his family. Although this woman could remarry, as it turned out she did not want to divorce the husband. She loved her family, and especially did not want to lose custody of her daughters. The point, of course, is that the woman's reproductive choice not to bear and rear additional children was overridden by other values she held simultaneously: love for her family and unwillingness to lose custody of her children.

This case was presented as having happened a long time ago. I asked whether it could still happen today, and was told "yes, in some remote mountainous areas." Remote mountainous areas are ostensibly the places where traditional Chinese values of women's husbands and mothers-in-law still rule the family.

Yet even long-held, traditional values undergo change. Today in China there is greater acceptance of (or adherence to) the "one family, one child" policy in cities than in the rural areas. I asked why this is so. In answer to my question, the following factors were mentioned:

1. People in the cities are more educated.
2. In rural areas there is nothing else for women to do besides have children and tend to the household.
3. In the countryside people have much more traditional values.
4. In the countryside people do not value education very much.
5. Under recently initiated policies, the peasants are getting rich, so now they surely see no need for better education since they can become wealthy without becoming educated.
6. A system of incentives in place in the city does not operate in the countryside.

Government's Role in Population Control

The last item mentioned above—the incentive system used by the Chinese government to limit family size—is a prominent example of the role governments have played in countries where population control policies have been instituted. Those policies can be highly influential in determining people's reproductive decisions and actions. An obstetrician/gynecologist from Shanghai characterized as an ongoing controversial issue in China the government decree that population growth must be reduced. Despite this government policy and its coercive methods of enforcement, there remains a traditional attitude that the government should not be involved in this way. I asked, "Who holds this view?" Her answer, "People who do not want to be limited. Their view is 'I want children; I want to have sons; the government should not limit me.'" This illustrates how traditional cultural values can influence reproductive choices even when severe penalties are attached to violation of government policies.

In contrast, a Beijing physician contended that most women want to limit births. The government pays for contraceptives, so the people get them free of charge. This is because of the high priority the government sets on limiting population growth, since the state does not pay for other medical services in China. The Beijing physician said that women are given a choice of contraceptive methods in the cities, but not in the countryside. The reason she cited was twofold: first, the difference in education between rural and urban women; and second, the efficacy of the methods used in the countryside. The physician said that in rural areas "women can't do family planning well by themselves. The woman may forget to take pills. And men don't want to use condoms."

The use of contraceptives in rural areas of China is thus dictated by what is made available to couples by the family planning commission, rather than by the cultural values of the people. The situation in China appears to be a complex mixture of coercive government policies, changing cultural values among urban and more educated people, and the desire of individual women to limit family size. In order to ascertain which of these factors determines the actual use of contraceptives, it is necessary to look at each case individually.

Another example taken from the Philippines is illustrative of the role of government. Under the long and repressive Marcos regime, family planning programs were established with the goal of reducing population growth.[11] Consistent with other practices under Marcos, coercive practices eventually became widespread, with some women being sterilized or having IUDs inserted without their knowledge and consent. Following the revolution and with the installation of Corazon Aquino as president of the Philippines, the extensive network of family planning services ground to a halt. This was largely due to the power and influence of the Catholic Church in the Philippines, and the fact that the Church supported Aquino's ascendancy to power. As a devout Catholic herself, Aquino appeared willing to go along with the Catholic Church's indifference to or active opposition of birth control.

As described by a nun who is a women's health advocate, the family planning program carried out during the years of the Marcos regime in the Philippines was coercive. In many cases IUDs were inserted in women without their knowledge and consent. After Marcos, the pendulum swung from coercive to nothing. The nun expressed her view that both extremes represent a violation of women's reproductive rights. It is evident that governmental policies, as well as cultural values, have been a leading determinant of contraceptive use in the Philippines.

Public Policy, Providers' Actions, and Social Class

The main argument of this paper is that freedom to choose a contraceptive method is influenced by cultural values, but ultimately determined by some combination of public policy and the behavior of medical personnel in hospitals or clinics. This section provides support for the second thesis stated at the outset: in developed as well as developing countries, the social and economic class to which a woman belongs, rather than cultural values, is what shapes the extent to which government policies and providers' actions affect a particular woman's use of contraceptives. China is probably a singular exception to this thesis, since the state's coercive power reaches into all classes of society.

In Mexico I attended a meeting with health sector personnel. One participant noted that in official documents, the right of the population to decide freely is taken for granted. For example, Article 4 of the Mexican Constitution asserts the right of each individual or couple to decide freely and responsibly on the number and spacing of their children. However, the assumption is made that because that right is stated in the law, it exists in reality. This participant asked, "What does this constitutional right mean in light of demographic goals in Mexico?" A basic problem stems from the fact that the issues are addressed at two different levels: the physician-patient relationship and policy implementation. Two related ethical questions emerge: (1) How can the reproductive rights of individuals be respected when goals for the acceptance of contraceptives are set by the government and imposed on each individual physician? (2) How can physicians maintain an ethical physician-patient relationship when pressure on them from the public family planning administration interferes with their clinical obligation to do what is best for the individual patient?

Two physicians at the meeting described poignantly and in detail the ethical dilemmas they face in their work in the public sector in Mexico. Beginning in their training, physicians are told to insert an IUD in every woman who has delivered three children. Since many women might refuse the IUD if asked, a large number of physicians insert the IUDs without informing women. One group of physicians was told to insert IUDs in women or else they would be fired from the hospital. Some of these doctors "complied" by inserting the IUDs in the women's vagina. The devices fell right out when the women stood up.

More subtle forms of coercion of women are also common. Contraceptives are commonly dealt with at the time the woman is in labor. This is held to be justified based on efficiency: to mount an educational program would otherwise be too costly. One physician referred to this as a "Third World method of coercion: the practice is held to be justified on the grounds that there are not enough resources to carry out the program in a more respectful way." Complicating matters further, placement of IUDs without the consent of the woman is, strictly speaking, illegal according to the dictates of Social Service (i.e., public) medical regulations. The Social Service practice is based on norms that require providing information to patients and gaining their consent. Yet a contradictory norm of this system requires physicians to place IUDs after childbirth or a Caesarean section. If a doctor does inform the woman about the IUD, it is when she is leaving the hospital.

Representatives of women's groups stated that an important value overlooked or denied to women in Mexico is freedom to choose. At present, both economic barriers and social controls militate against a woman's freedom to choose a preferred contraceptive method. For example, diaphragms are unavailable because they are viewed by physicians as an unreliable method.

Some physicians cite a study showing that Mexican women do not want to touch their genitals, and so physicians refuse even to offer diaphragms as a contraceptive method.

Not all means of family planning are acceptable to the population. One participant in a meeting suggested that if allowed a choice, women may select a method of contraception that carries a higher risk of pregnancy but has fewer side effects than a more effective method with undesirable side effects. She surmised that women would rather become pregnant than use a contraceptive method with side effects. She added that the population in Mexico does not want hormonal methods or IUDs, but these are the methods promoted by the family planning agency. Also noted was the fact that many rural women object to IUDs because they are opposed to placement of a foreign object in their bodies. It was stated that the three contraceptive methods most preferred by the population are sterilization, the rhythm method, and the condom.

However, as the system is structured, if couples accept the condom they do not officially count as "acceptors" by the administration that governs family planning policy. As an illustration of the systemic paternalism and lack of concern for women's own values, the remark of a marketer for Cyclofem was quoted: "This is a feminist method; what does it matter if it has side effects?"

In China, freedom to choose is a rare occurrence, despite the claim by one physician that all methods are usually available. This physician did acknowledge that in some regions of the country, a decision was made that the IUD is the best method because it does not require daily action by women. I asked the physician about hormonal methods, and he said that Norplant and DMPA are available in China, but women do not like these methods because they affect the menstrual cycle and cause bleeding.

A Shanghai physician also said that many contraceptive methods are in use all over the country, but there is poor follow-up. As a result, not much is known about what happens once family planning programs are implemented. In this physician's words, "Things have simply been done mechanically." As an example, she noted the stipulation that after having two children a woman should be sterilized. This practice is carried out even among women who have had an IUD inserted. For another example, women are told to have an IUD inserted after having one child. Even though the woman might prefer oral contraceptives to an IUD, she is not given that option because "she could not be trusted to take the pills regularly."

A controversy has arisen among physicians and others over the question of whether it is right to insist that all women use the same contraceptive. This Shanghai physician is among those who say "no," that contraceptive methods should be individualized to each woman. This is not something that should be done mechanically or uniformly, since some methods are better for one person, other methods for another.

A related issue is that of women not wanting to be sterilized after having two children, as the government policy requires. The IUD is removed and the woman is sterilized. As a result, women suffer psychologically. The Shanghai physician contended that this is wrong on two counts: first, it is medically contraindicated as "unnecessary surgery," since the IUD could remain in place and thereby prevent conception; second, the practice is wrong because it causes psychological harm to women. Her judgment that this practice is ethically wrong is based on its actual or potential bad consequences. As could be expected, this ethical issue in China is not framed in the language of rights—specifically, the rights of the individual—but in terms of harmful and beneficial consequences. This serves as a reminder that it is not necessary to use the language of rights in justifying claims about the ethics of a particular action or a general practice.

The implementation of coercive policies limiting choice varies from one country to another. As described earlier, physicians in Mexico are taught as part of their training to insert IUDs in women who have had three children. Some physicians fear penalties or loss of privileges for failure to comply. In China there is still not much in the way of current practice requiring informed consent. Family planning workers are the ones who have forced people to use IUDs or be sterilized. If a woman has one child, a daughter, she may want a son. But she is forced to take pills, have an IUD inserted, or be sterilized. I inquired what mechanism is used to force a woman to take birth control pills. A Chinese bioethicist said that the system is highly developed: a worker can come to the home and insist on observing women taking their pills. If a woman goes ahead and has a second child, she will have to pay the penalty. The local family planning worker decides what that penalty shall be.

Third-World Coercion in the United States

In the United States, the federal government, state governments, and the judiciary have both sought and gained the authority to exert controls, direct or indirect, over the reproductive lives of some citizens, either individually or as members of a class. That control can range from court-ordered procedures (e.g., Caesarean sections, detention of pregnant women in hospitals, and mandates to obey doctors' orders) to issuing alternative sentences to a jail term (e.g., acceptance of Norplant insertion), to legislative attempts to provide monetary incentives to welfare recipients if they accept Norplant.

Although this country is multicultural and cultural values can influence the contraceptive choices of women, whatever ethical problems have arisen with long-term contraception do not appear to stem from the phenomenon of multiculturalism. Rather, in the United States as in other countries, ethical concerns can be traced more to social class than to membership in an ethnic or racial minority group. Attempts by policymakers to control the fertility of some women by means of long-term contraceptives fall disproportionately on the poor. As a consequence, there is bound to be a differential impact on ethnic and racial minorities when such groups constitute a substantial proportion of the poorer classes in society. In the United States, to the extent that African-Americans, Native Americans, and Latinas are poor, less well educated, or receiving welfare payments, they are likely to be among the main targets of reproductive control. Middle-class and better educated blacks, Native Americans, and Hispanics have as much (or as little) in the way of reproductive freedoms as white women, so differences in cultural beliefs and practices do not pose a problem vis-a-vis dominant or mainstream cultural values.

There is, however, one important difference between the government's role in the United States and in developing countries where policies have been introduced regarding long-term contraceptives. Those countries are in varying degrees poor, but more important, they have a serious if not an urgent problem of population growth. That problem does not exist in the United States. Reducing population growth in developing countries has been seen as necessary for sustaining a reasonable quality of life for the population as a whole, and also for preventing eventual widespread famine and severe pressure on other resources.

However, it has recently become a matter of considerable controversy whether government restrictions on fertility are the only or even the most effective way of reducing population growth in developing countries. The correlation between development and decline of fertility is a phenomenon in every country, and the educational level of women has been shown to be a significant factor associated with a reduction in the number of children per family.

Unlike those developing countries with a population growth problem, the United States is highly developed, rich, and does not exhibit a demographic pattern of too-rapid population growth threatening the well-being of the nation as a whole. One can only conclude, then, that the motives of politicians and other policymakers regarding Norplant are narrowly economic and broadly political, designed to save middle-class and wealthy taxpayers money by targeting welfare recipients for public policy involving Norplant. The concern in the United States is money and the unwillingness of the taxpayers to pay for poor people's babies.

A Cautionary Tale: Values of the Health Care Provider

The following case illustrates the thesis that the values of the health care provider also play a role, one that can readily override the values of the less powerful patient. This is especially true following an increase in the variety of long-term contraceptives, enabling physicians to control women's fertility in accordance with the physicians' values. The legal and ethical requirements for physicians to obtain informed consent, along with the generally higher educational level of women and their ability to assert their autonomy more effectively, makes limitations on reproductive freedom in the clinical setting less likely to occur in the United States than in many developing countries. Nevertheless, here is a cautionary tale.

A physician brought the following case to the hospital ethics committee. The patient was a 30-year-old mildly mentally retarded woman. One year earlier, the woman had come to the hospital seeking an abortion. At that time the patient was living with her mother. The patient had had consensual sex with her boyfriend, but they were not married and had since broken up. Psychiatrists evaluated her and found her competent to consent to the abortion on her own behalf. She understood that she was pregnant, that the abortion would terminate the pregnancy, what the risks and benefits of the procedure were, and that her alternative was to carry the pregnancy to term. The woman signed consent for the procedure, and her mother also signed. The physician raised the subject of inserting a Norplant implant during the same informed consent discussion for the abortion. Again, the patient was said to understand the relevant information in order to grant informed consent. The physician told her that Norplant remained effective for five years. The woman was being urged by her mother to accept the Norplant, so there was some question about the voluntariness of her consent. Nevertheless, having been judged competent to consent, she was entitled to receive the Norplant. The physician performed the abortion and inserted the Norplant.

One year later the patient returned to the clinic, requesting that the Norplant be removed. She had reunited with her former boyfriend (the man by whom she had become pregnant), and they were now married. She said she wanted a child. She was 30 years old, saw women around her having babies, and said she and her husband very much wanted to have a child. The woman's husband was also mildly mentally retarded. They lived together in their own apartment, which they were able to maintain adequately. Both were being supported financially by the city and state.

The physician was unwilling to remove the Norplant. He brought the case to the hospital ethics committee because, he said, he was being criticized by other staff. He said he was "conscientiously opposed" to removing the Norplant and believed that he was therefore not required to do so. By way of analogy, the doctor contended that if health professionals could refuse to participate in abortions on the grounds of moral conscience, so too could he refuse to remove Norplant based on similar considerations.

The physician gave three reasons for his "conscientious refusal" to remove the Norplant:

1. The woman and her husband were mentally retarded, and so there was a question of whether they could adequately care for and raise a child.

2. The woman had been informed that a Norplant implant was effective for five years. She had consented to its insertion—therefore, she consented to having it in place for five years, and the physician was not required to remove it.

3. If they did have a child, it would cost the state even more money than the support already being given to the couple. If they kept the baby, they would need some sort of home health aide; if they were forced to relinquish the child because of inability to care for it, that too would cost the state money.

The first reason given by the physician may well be a legitimate ethical concern, but that concern is not one that authorizes physicians to make unilateral reproductive decisions on behalf of patients. The long, ignoble history of sterilizing people judged to be mentally retarded should serve as a reminder of how readily doctors contributed to a practice now widely held to constitute an abuse of reproductive rights. Although a long-acting contraceptive like Norplant or an IUD has the advantage of reversibility, it is still necessary to have a skilled clinician available to remove the contraceptive if the patient requests it. This physician was unwilling to do so.

The second reason given by the doctor reveals his misunderstanding of the process of informed consent. He argued that since he told the patient that Norplant was effective for five years and she consented to insertion of the implant, he was under no obligation to her to remove it before the five-year period was over. Either the physician omitted telling the patient that even though the implant would be effective for five years, that did not mean she had to keep it in for that long; or he did inform her but refused nonetheless to remove it at her request. In either case, the physician failed in his obligation to the patient. As the ethics committee eventually concluded, if this physician is unwilling to remove Norplant from any patient he should not insert the implant in the first place. The committee also questioned the timing of the consent discussion, since it took place at the same time the patient was consenting to undergo an abortion.

The third reason given by the physician brings us to the heart of the matter. This physician, along with a growing number of doctors in our country, views himself as an agent of society with a greater obligation to taxpayers than to his patients. In this case, it was the mental retardation of the patient and her husband that led to the doctor's supposition that the couple would need public support to help rear the child. However, this same physician had on a subsequent occasion told the ethics committee that numerous women in whom he had inserted Norplant were "abusing the system" by requesting removal within months after the implantation. The women's reason in this latter group of cases was their inability to tolerate the side effects of Norplant. The committee wondered whether the physician had adequately informed the patients in advance of the likelihood of side effects and the varying degrees of severity such effects could have in different women. Of course, even if he did properly inform these patients in advance, the women still retain the right to have the Norplant removed once they actually experience the side effects.

No information was provided about the race or ethnicity of the mentally retarded woman or the group of women who requested removal of the Norplant because of the side effects. But it is clear that all are poor, all are users of the city hospital system, and it is likely that few or none have private insurance. The physician made quite clear his belief that these women are costing society too much money by first consenting to receive the expensive Norplant and then requesting to have the implant removed. He also made clear his personal view that the retarded couple should not be having children. From other evidence in the hospital (unrelated to these Norplant cases), it is known that the physician holds the view that poor women who come to the city hospital are "irresponsibly" having too many children. He appears to see it as part of his job to counter their irresponsible behavior by seeking to ensure that they accept Norplant and keep it in place.

Conclusion

This physician is not unique in his attitudes and beliefs. Examples of similar values are cited in the report entitled "Creating Ethical Reproductive Health Care Policy: Views and Values Concerning Norplant."[12] Letters to Ann Landers expressed opinions about a welfare system that "rewards unwed mothers with cash for each child," with readers stating that "forced birth control is the only solution" and that "these irresponsible brood mares should be sterilized after the second baby."[13]

Also revealing but misguided in another respect is the statement attributed to one health care provider: "What's wrong with incentives? It's offering a prize to someone for doing something."[14] The notion that providing incentives to poor women not to have children is like offering a prize to someone who does something meritorious contains a peculiar distortion. What if we substituted the word "bribe" for "prize"? It would then seem much less like a monetary prize awarded for an accomplishment and more like a bribe to a person not to do something that others would prefer her not to do.

Although the differences between the United States and developing countries are greater than the similarities when it comes to policies and practices relating to long-term contraception, one strand of similarity stands out: the selection in every society of poor or disadvantaged women as targets for policies aimed at controlling their fertility.

One U.S. policymaker was quoted as saying, "We pay farmers not to grow crops. . . ."[15] This analogy between paying women to accept Norplant and paying farmers not to grow crops reveals a remarkable assumption about women and human reproduction. It suggests that the relationship between a woman and her reproductive capacity is the same as that between a farmer and his land. It implies that the reason women have children is similar to the reason farmers grow crops. And it utterly fails to acknowledge the physical side effects of the method employed to get the woman not to grow babies, effects that have no analogy to the farmer. Treating women as targets of population control policies is a well-known phenomenon in developing countries. Proposed policies and attempts to use the courts in the service of controlling women's fertility suggest that these Third World methods are gaining favor in the United States. In a country where people get paid for not producing commodities, it is becoming acceptable to pay women for not having children.

Seeking to save taxpayers money by using financial incentives to control the fertility of poor women is a "Third World" method of coercion. Enlisting doctors to serve the interests of the state in saving society money or in meting out judicial punishments for child abuse treats physicians as instruments of government policies rather than as agents of their patients. As developing countries become more like the United States in their economic systems and the availability of material goods, the United States is becoming more like them in the use of state policies to control women's reproductive choices. Two decades of activity by states and the federal government to erode women's right to abortion is one example of this. The flurry of activity in courts and legislatures following the introduction of Norplant is another.

Ethical objections to the array of activities noted above do not rest on considerations of autonomy and liberty alone. Also involved are considerations of justice, since neither in the United States nor in other countries have educated and economically advantaged women been coerced or offered incentives to be sterilized or to be "acceptors" of long-term contraceptives. If the second thesis propounded here is accurate—that the social and economic class to which a woman belongs, rather than cultural values, is what shapes the extent to which government policies and providers' actions affect a particular woman's use of contraceptives—then justice-based obligations are central to the ethical analysis.

So long as women or couples have the information, the opportunity, and the means to freely choose among alternative modes of contraception, the values or norms of the culture to which they belong are likely to be less influential than their individual preferences. Women and couples may reject the traditional values or prescribed rules of a group to which they otherwise adhere—as, for example, do those Roman Catholics the world over who ignore the church's prohibition against artificial contraception.

Whether it stems from religious, cultural, or other traditional roots, the value of having children is fundamental in every society. That value is perfectly compatible with the desire of individuals or couples not to have any children or to limit their families to one child. Control over one's reproductive life is a salient value that marks the line over which the government should not step in its efforts to reduce welfare payments or to mete out punishments in the criminal justice system. Policymakers and health care providers in the United States should thus avoid the missteps of government officials and family planning workers in developing countries. Long-term contraceptives must not be used to serve the interests of the state, but rather to provide optimal reproductive health services to the population.

NOTES

1. Miho Ogino, "Japanese Women and the Decline of the Birth Rate," *Reproductive Health Matters*, no. 1 (1993): 79.

2. FINRRAGE opposes reproductive technology in general and IVF techniques in particular. This radical feminist group holds that such technologies represent the newest effort by men to control women. Different groups specifically oppose hormonal methods. See, for example, Barbara Mintzes, Anita Hardon, and Jannemieke Hanhart, eds., *Norplant: Under Her Skin* (Amsterdam: Eburon, Women's Health Action Foundation, 1993).

3. Segun Gbadegesin, "Bioethics and Culture: An African Perspective," *Bioethics* 7, no. 2/3 (1993): 258.

4. Supported by a grant from the Ford Foundation, I visited these three countries from 1992 to 1993 as part of a project on ethics and reproductive health. Throughout this article, observations and quotations are based on information I gathered in interviews and meetings during these visits.

5. Ren-Zong Qiu, "Morality in Flux: Medical Ethics Dilemmas in the People's Republic of China," *Kennedy Institute of Ethics Journal* 1 (1991): 16–17.

6. Qiu, "Morality in Flux," 18.

7. *New York Times*, 4 August 1993. A11.

8. This recommendation for correct terminology has been made by Rebecca Cook, an expert on international reproductive rights who is on the faculty of law at the University of Toronto.

9. Maria del Carmen Elu, "Abortion Yes, Abortion No, in Mexico," *Reproductive Health Matters*, no. 1 (1993): 59.

10. Elu, "Abortion Yes, Abortion No," 59.

11. Donald P. Warwick, *Bitter Pills: Population Policies and Their Implementation in Eight Developing Countries* (Cambridge: Cambridge University Press, 1982), 17–19.

12. Cheri Pies, *Creating Ethical Reproductive Health Care Policy: Views and Values Concerning Norplant* (n.p., n.d.).

13. Pies, *Norplant*, 9.

14. Pies, *Norplant*, 26.

15. Pies, *Norplant*, 26.

TOLA OLU PEARCE

Ethical Issues in the Importation of Long-Acting Contraceptives to Nigeria

Nigeria is a former British colony which received its independence in 1960. It is said to be the most ethnically diverse nation in Africa with over three hundred ethnic groups and is recognized as the third largest multilingual nation in the world. Its history has been dominated by ethnic rivalry, much of which was fuelled by the colonial administration. Nigeria's population dynamics have become front page news, but demographic information has remained scanty and much of the data are controversial. Most censuses conducted this century have been rejected as unreliable. Even the 1963 census was accepted as a political compromise. In 1991, the census was again taken, but has yet to be officially accepted due to the same ethno-political wranglings which plagued earlier censuses. Extrapolating from the 1963 figures (55.6 million), Nigeria is said to have a population of between 100 and 126 million. However, the preliminary figures for the 1991 census put the size at 88.5 million.[1] But the population statistics about which the government is now concerned are the annual growth rate and the total fertility rate (TFR). While the former is above 3% per annum, the latter is 6.[2] After a long period of refusing to pay attention to population growth rates, the government presently holds the view that rapid growth rates impede development. The ongoing debate revolves around the role poverty plays in keeping the TFR high or the role a high TFR plays in economic stagnation. The government endorses the latter thesis. Unfortunately, Nigeria's low standard of living cannot be denied. But there are many who support the first thesis. Nonetheless, the life expectancy is still only fifty-two years, the infant mortality rate in 1991 was 86 per 1,000, and the maternal mortality rate (in excess of 1,000 per 100,000) is believed to be one of the highest in Africa.[3] The Society of Obstetricians and Gynecologists (SOLON) reported in 1990 that a woman dies every ten minutes from pregnancy and related problems.[4]

Since the 1950s, the international population establishment has focussed its attention on linking population growth to lack of development in Third World nations. After 1960, attention was specifically turned to Africa and a number of African nations, including Egypt, Kenya, and Ghana, inaugurated national population policies to control growth rates. The population scholars argue that rapid population growth rates impede economic development by accelerating consumption, slowing savings or investments, and reducing the resources available for development projects (e.g., education, health, welfare services). With the downward spiral in the standard of living in the 1980s and external encouragement, the Nigerian government reconsidered its long-standing lack of interest in population control.

A National Population Policy was developed in 1988 and implemented in 1989.[5] On the whole, the policy is a comprehensive outline of the direction activities need to take for an improvement in the quality of life of the populace. It targets population size, the growth rate, infertility, inequalities in health status, and imbalances in urban/rural population distribution as requiring attention. It does, however, express the hope that the growth rate will be reduced to 2% and the TFR to four children per female by the year 2000.[6] With these targets, the focus of implementation has been overwhelmingly on the distribution of modern contraceptives among women. It has been open season for both government and nongovernment (NGOs) family planning schemes and contraception experiments across the nation.[7] Married women in the rural areas are the main focus of interest, since by the age of nineteen, about 83% of Nigerian females are married and 65% of the population resides in the rural areas.[8] But increasingly, there is speculation over how best to develop programs aimed specifically at the adolescent population.[9]

The use of fertility-regulating methods is indigenous to local communities in Nigeria. Both long-acting and short-term contraceptive techniques evolved during the precolonial area. There are various indigenous herbal mixtures taken orally as well as other magical and nonmagical procedures. Amulets, waistbands, and rings are often viewed as magical as are other rituals such as the one in which locked padlocks are secretly buried by the indigenous healer who is then required at a latter date to unlock the padlock (unlock the womb). However, it was pointed out to me by researchers of the Obafemi Awolowo University pharmacy faculty that some of these rings had been soaked in liquid compounds. The questions are: do some chemicals seep into the skin when the rings are worn, and is this effective? These still remain unanswered questions. Nonetheless, contraceptives—as a subgroup of fertility regulating techniques—were developed for spacing or to safeguard the health of infants, and terminal abstinence signaled the onset of maternal grandparenthood.[10] Today, much of this indigenous knowledge has been lost, and all methods, with the exception of abstinence, have been officially declared as "inefficient" techniques. The present interest in reducing the rate of population growth therefore focuses on Western (modern) imported techniques. Imported contraceptives became available in the late 1950s, but acceptance was slow, and government interest was lukewarm, as already noted.[11] The Nigerian Fertility Survey reports that in the early 1980s only one-tenth of the 6% of women using a method of family planning were using modern contraceptives.[12] Subsequent to the 1988 Population Policy, Nigeria was drawn into the circle of Third World nations importing large quantities of Western contraceptive techniques.

In the West, the bulk of resources for research on contraception have been allocated to developing long-acting surgical or hormonal (female) methods since the 1960s,[13] even though some attention has been turned to various barrier methods as a result of the AIDS pandemic. In Nigeria, the pill, IUDs, Depo-Provera, and sterilization are now available. Noristerat is being used on an experimental basis, but abortion is still illegal. It is not inconceivable that a female vaccine will be introduced once it is accepted internationally as an efficient method. In 1993, such a vaccine was proposed for testing in a number of countries including India and Kenya.[14] Of the methods regularly available in Nigeria, the pill, IUDs, and Depo-Provera appear to be popular in that order. The resistance to sterilization has been substantial.

Framework for Review of Ethical Issues

In order to review the ethical issues surrounding the importation and use of long-acting Western contraceptives in Nigeria, I propose a breakdown into three levels: (1) the *global*; (2) *national*; and (3) *household* levels. While each of these three tiers will be discussed separately, the interaction between these and its overall impact cannot be ignored and will also be highlighted. First, at the global level it is important to understand the ways in which Nigeria's position within the world economic system has influenced the focus of the population concerns. On the national level, questions need to be asked about the role played by local experts and professionals in the population control debate. Finally, we need to turn to the micro-level of communities and households and review power and gender struggles over the use of contraceptives within the extended family.

Family planning services in Nigeria received a boost not only from the development of the Population Policy, but also from the inauguration of the Primary Health Care (PHC) program which became the bedrock of the 1988 National Health Care Policy. Maternal and child health (MCH) services were one of the nine dimensions of PHC, and family planning was to be an integral part of each MCH clinic.[15] Initially, the country was divided into four health zones, and various institutions—including the federal government, UNICEF, and schools of technology—were given a free hand in developing model PHC services which could later be incorporated into a national PHC system. Under this arrangement, long-acting contraceptives were to be introduced into local communities and advertised as a health measure for reducing the incidence of infant and maternal mortality emanating from rapid and prolonged child-bearing.

Gender Politics at the Household and Community Levels

One fallout from polygyny has been the competition between wives to produce offspring. This includes the battle between "inside" and "outside" wives.[16] All categories of "wives" attempt to stake their claim on a relationship by producing children for the man, his extended family, and lineage. In the tensions that develop in a home, middle-class men have been known to declare a moratorium on childbearing by the wife at home, only to proceed to have additional children outside. In this tussle, long-acting contraceptives (notably sterilization) are implicated, and women are well aware of their vulnerability in this regard. Furthermore, we must question the ethics of pressing for sterilization in an environment in which infant mortality rates remain unaccept-ably high. On the reverse side of gender power dynamics within households, women have at times attempted to control their fertility in the face of male and extended family opposition. Therefore some have sought contraception secretly. Initially when the husband's signature or presence at the clinic was required as evidence of consent, women made use of male relatives or friends. Long-acting methods such as Depo-Provera—and to a lesser extent, the pill—became useful. These allow a woman to act independently of the wishes of a man or his family.

The contraceptive safety issue has become a major concern of women's groups both inside and outside Nigeria.[17] Ogbuagu reports how Depo-Provera is sold over the counter in Nigeria and even along the roadside, as are many prescription drugs owing to the laxity in regulations. The focus on efficiency and massive distribution among the populace exposes women to questionable practices and health risks, as these drugs filter through the various distribution systems (both legal and illegal). In a forthcoming article based on material gathered from a couple of model PHC family planning service centers in the late 1980s, I reported on the lack of equipment for examination and follow-up among "acceptors."[18] More recent data from 147 family planning service delivery points (SDP) in six states (covering all the four health divisions of Nigeria) confirm these findings. Mensch et al. concluded that "[i]n Nigeria, the conditions for aseptic services are lacking in many facilities: only 37 percent have disposable gloves and slightly more than half (56 percent) have adequate water."[19] In addition, only 41% have sterilizing lotion and 45% have sterilizers. It was also noted that one-quarter of SDPs with adequate water were not clean. While only 6% of the staff lacked basic training in family planning, records were frequently not kept either because the SDP staff "did not know how to or were simply uninterested . . . Indeed, in order to produce the data on a number of family planning visits that were made to several service-delivery points, the Nigerian field teams had to organize and compile the records themselves."[20] From this study, it appears that more attention has been paid to the availability of commodities (pill, IUD, injectables, etc.) than to other material known to be crucial for maintaining the health of clients.

Again, according to Dixon-Mueller, service delivery within the population control rhetoric follows the "inoculation mentality" in which too much emphasis is placed on providing single antipregnancy "shots" such as IUDs, injections, and implants rather than on the health consequences of these methods.[21] All those health risk concerns which scholars in North America have enumerated, particularly those dealing with hormonal methods, must necessarily apply to African women. Thus, with regard to women's bodies, long-acting contraceptives may have short-term (e.g., nausea, spotting, headaches) and long-term (e.g., thrombosis, cancer) health consequences.

The Nation: Ethical Responsibilities of Professionals

As a result of Western education and colonization, a wide range of professional and paraprofessional groups now work in the modern health sector outside of the indigenous enclave. These include physicians and other health care providers such as nurses and additional staff in family planning clinics, lawyers, social scientists, social workers, and various therapists. Many are involved in research (basic and applied scientific studies) on the distribution of contraceptives. Since independence, numerous strategies have been advocated for development, and health development has become the latest in a string of attempts to improve the desperate situation. Therefore, since the mid-1980s, work in health research has escalated. At the same time, interest in the ethical responsibilities of professionals in health has grown.

The growth of professional groups has been a mixed blessing in all societies. Abbot reminds us about the power over laypersons, monopoly of rewards/resources, and control over knowledge production that comes with the rise of professional groups.[22] Thus Western scholars are divided over the balance between benefits and the price that attends the professionalization of society.[23] All professional groups are confronted with an overwhelming number of ethical issues ranging from the most personal to the visibly public. They interact with various categories of "alters" in their daily work. These include peers and others in the institutional work place, the government, the society (or public at large), individual clients or research subjects, and foreign sponsors/ agencies. Ethical standards are implicated in all these relationships which are too numerous to consider all at once in this short essay. Discussion will, therefore, be restricted to two groups: the society at large and clients (or research subjects).

With regard to the public, professionals in Nigeria operate in a context where only 50 percent (60 percent male, 40 percent female) of the population is literate. The educational gap between most professionals and others remains wide, unlike in many Western societies. This calls into question the degree of accountability emanating from the public. The Western system of health care is not bound by the old methods of accountability developed for health care practitioners within the indigenous sector. Nonetheless, like other professionals worldwide, their acquisition of knowledge and technical expertise, according to Jennings et al., demand that attention be paid to two modes of service.[24] Professionals are responsible to the nation for pursuing the public interest and opening up relevant debates on the common good. The duty to promote the public interest "includes the professions' contribution of technical expertise to public policy analysis. . . ."[25] Professionals help forge the direction of public policy by working through associations, conferences, and their private publications. In Nigeria policymakers and advisers have generally included professionals. As Ayodele argues, "professionals . . . join the civil service as technical officers who provide information and ideas, most of which are required on technical matters such as technology, economics, medicine, engineering, statistics, etc. . . . The bulk of policy decisions of the government are made by [the] civil servants in collaboration with the professionals."[26] Nigeria has had a tradition, in the postindependence era, of calling on professionals in the universities, polytechnics, and research institutes to brainstorm and provide advice on any pressing issue. Ayodele goes on to criticize the tendency to "simply give the impression of situations of the non-availability of alternatives in order to create monopolistic conditions around favored choices. Under such situations, sub-optimal policy-decisions would be made."[27] He hints at the problems that occur when professionals merely serve as "rubber-stamps," endorsing and pushing policies through. Often institutional reorganization has been suggested to deal with this problem. But does this reach the heart of the matter?

In turning attention specifically to the population debate and community experiments with long-acting contraceptives, we need to delve into the advisory role played by different groups of professionals. In reviewing their activities, it would also be incumbent on the researcher to understand the subjective experience of professionals and their personal responses to opportunities and constraints. How are incoming concepts and projects evaluated? For instance, *popular participation* was the buzzword of the 1980s. However, studies indicate that its popularity did not alter the fact that the concept remains ambiguous and ill-defined in Nigeria. Community participation has meant different things to different people,[28] and as Olowu[29] correctly pointed out, getting communities involved may be cosmetic: mere decentralization for the purpose of reducing the cost of implementing a program rather than developing self-governance. Furthermore, studies have revealed that in health care programs, community participation is the weakest link in program development.[30]

In seeking to promote the common good, professionals must bring their unique knowledge to bear on debates about "basic human values, and on facets of the human good and the good life. It also includes the professions' contribution to what may be called civic discourse or public philosophy."[31] In a country such as Nigeria, this would entail initiating the debate on the interaction between Western and indigenous values as they influence our conceptions of a good (great?) society. Such debates would focus on institution building (values, meanings, and practices) and the type of society we want in the future. With respect to health and population growth, concerns turn to discussions of what constitutes good health and the most effective building blocks for a healthy population. Conferences on technology transfer (e.g., contraceptives) in the absence of a broad understanding of health invite failure.

For the most part, good health has been equated "with the provision of a physician and a hospital"[32] rather than with public health facilities (clean water, refuse disposal) or community decision making in health issues, cheaper foodstuffs, higher income, more education, etc. The meager health budget has generally been spent on curative as opposed to preventive care, and health is seen as a "medical" problem. One must, however, admit that criticisms of this approach date back more than twenty years.[33] There have been many conferences in Nigeria at which some physician stands up to remind participants that clean, pipe-borne water will presently save more lives than expensive imported drugs. At this point, we need to go beyond rhetoric to uncover the danger points—i.e., the points at which such knowledge is blocked rather than being translated into action. One needs to query the ethics of encouraging the prompt distribution of long-acting hormonal contraceptives at a time when other services are shrinking and user fees have been reintroduced. This seems to be a problem presently faced by women throughout Africa.[34]

Professional responsibilities to research subjects and clinic clients are many, but interest in the doctrine of *informed consent* has perhaps caught the greatest attention. The right of the research subject or client to know all the risks and benefits resulting from the intervention in which he/she is about to participate and the need to give consent are at the core of this doctrine. These rights and duties are often interpreted differently within different societies—the role of cultural relativity is therefore now being seriously debated internationally. For instance, in America the doctrine operates within the context of a culture that is rights-oriented. Notions of self-determination, autonomy, and consumer choice take precedence over all else.[35] England, a nation without a written constitution, has had a long history of a more paternalistic relationship between clients and professionals in which the duties of the latter are emphasized. Thus a physician is given more leeway in deciding what is reasonable for a patient to know or to consume during treatment. In addition, the class kinship between the older professions helps maintain a united front vis-à-vis the public.[36]

Questions have been asked about Africa now that research projects and development programs have become commonplace. Will a cultural context in which the individual is embedded in the social group (collectivist orientation) alter the meaning or process of obtaining informed consent? Maybe, but this cannot be decided until after open debate within each separate African nation. Serious debates will include—but not be limited to—suggestions and statements from professionals. Some scholars believe that because of the relational definition of personhood and the traditional authority of local leaders, consent should be sought only from these intermediaries at the community or household levels.[37] But also, both a first-person and a community authority consent procedure has been suggested.

As part of the debate, a number of issues need to be brought forward. The first is that even though privacy and individualism may be weak concepts in Africa, *individuality* is well recognized.[38] Also, within Nigeria, the various subcultures may perceive issues differently and one ethnic perspective cannot be imposed on all. During the debate aimed at a national policy or perspective, different voices will need to be heard. In addition, we must take into account the fact that with medical interventions such as long-acting contraception, an individual's physical body will, in the final analysis, bear the brunt. When dealing with whose interest comes first, we need to be wary of arguments which state that in Africa "it is difficult to see how the interests of the subject conflict with the interests of society, except, of course, if the society is not his own."[39] Many ethnic groups emphasize hierarchy in conjunction with collectivism. Those at the bottom of the hierarchy (e.g., young females) are expected to bear a disproportionate share of the group's trauma. Is this something we wish to perpetuate, even if it can be shown to be indigenous?

Ijsselmuiden and Faden have argued convincingly that proposals to modify informed consent procedures in Africa must be thoroughly scrutinized.[40] Questionable reasons include the following:

Lower costs, lower risks of litigation, less stringent ethical reviews, the availability of populations prepared to cooperate with almost any study that appears curative in nature, anticipated under reporting of side effects because of low consumer awareness, the desire for personal advancement, and the desire to create new markets for pharmaceutical agents and other products.[41]

Politically, the social body of Africa has been the most penetrated on the globe and this has had long-term effects on the way physical bodies are handled. Nigerian professionals must be alert to our position in the status-craving contemporary culture of Nigeria.[42] More serious discussion is needed before we can decide whether it is informed or uninformed consent which is required, under what conditions, and with respect to whom.[43]

The International Impact

The importation of long-acting contraceptives has become part of the broader process of development management, instigated from outside but involving numerous layers of external and internal actors. At the global level, the population control debate is informed by a number of perspectives including the conservative, liberal, and Marxist perspectives.[44] In contradiction to what often appears as a monolithic viewpoint which attaches growth rates to lack of development and rapid resource consumption, there has in fact been much disagreement. Simon even goes as far as to argue that "in the 1980s a revolution occurred in scientific views about the effect of population growth on economic development: economists stopped asserting that population increases must exhaust natural resources and preclude economic growth . . . The lack of news of this revolution is itself newsworthy."[45] Thus, according to Simon, little has actually changed in reporting by the popular press and among program developers. By the end of the 1980s, the consistent pressure exerted on specific nations had the intended impact.

The ethical import of this scenario has not, however, escaped the attention of several scholars. One question hinges on the problems associated with global pressures within a hierarchical world economic system in which some nations set the context for debate and define what are to be regarded as "urgent" problems, the methods to be employed for arriving at such statements, and the type of national solutions to be sought. Specific to demographic issues, there has developed what Riedmann refers to in her recent book, entitled *Science That Colonizes,* as the World System Demography.[46]

Riedmann draws attention to the fact that the contemporary population control debate and methods of marshalling information are part of a long history of interaction between the West and Third World nations. The pattern was set centuries ago. She argues that "the authority of First World scientists to penetrate Third World areas for the purpose of gathering information is a carryover from the 'right-to-invade' established in the fifteenth century and thereafter by musket-bearing Europeans."[47] In this latest round of activities, data are carted out and knowledge constructed to control the area. In *Science That Colonizes*, Riedmann draws on fertility studies conducted in the 1970s in southwest Nigeria in order to focus on the ways in which family planning necessarily comes with a large cultural package, including an underlying devaluation of indigenous knowledge; a covert premise that locals cannot solve their problems; the introduction of specific world views about the ideal nature of children (or the family); and the use of local staff to break down resistance among the research subjects by the employment of "cultural capital" to win respondents over. As the economic situation worsens, with unemployment and underemployment on the rise, we can expect many more educated people to be available for such work. Data on contraceptive prevalence, practices and outcomes will be a major industry for some time.

It is also true that once the markets for contraceptive commodities have been developed, the road is open for continuous profit for foreign companies. According to Alubo, African nations have become increasingly dependent on imported drugs.[48] With the exception of Egypt and South Africa, dependence is about 80% on the continent. The present trends in the use of long-acting contraceptives are part of this process.

Conclusion

This chapter is not about rejecting the idea of contraception for women (and men), nor about denying the importance of making long-term contraceptives available in Nigeria. It is about the context—ideological and programmatic—within which these commodities are introduced on a wide scale. Many Nigerians have become concerned about the emphasis of the National Population Policy, the numerous distribution programs, and the inattention to the health and control dimensions of policy implementation. Both the government and professionals are implicated in the way these services are developed and carried out among women, especially the rural poor.

Medical research on Third World women has become a sensitive issue. There is yet to develop any serious debate and consensus on the work of researchers in Nigeria. Each is generally left to his/her conscience and possesses some general knowledge that client or patient consent is in order. A lot of this research involves the testing of imported techniques. It has been argued that Nigeria, along with many other African countries, does not have the resources to develop new techniques. Yet there is always the option of regional collaboration and the development of indigenously based methods. None of the most efficient methods used in the West today would have reached such stages of refinement without the amount of financial nurturing they received. While there are a few institutions where indigenous contraceptive research is being conducted (e.g., Obafemi Awolowo University, Ife), funding is pitiful.

In summary, this chapter reveals how the importation of long-acting contraceptives touches on all levels of the political and economic lives of Nigerians, from the health of female bodies to the relationship of Nigeria to international groups and foreign governments.

NOTES

1. Federal Government of Nigeria, *1991 Population Census: Provisional Results* (Lagos: Government Printer. 1992), 1.

2. Federal Ministry of Health, Department of Population Activities, *National Policy on Population for Development, Unity, Progress and Self-Reliance* (Lagos: Government Printer, 1988), 3–4.

3. United Nations Children's Fund (UNICEF), *The State of the World's Children*, (Oxford: Oxford University Press, 1993), 68, 80.

4. Society of Obstetricians and Gynecologists of Nigeria (SOLON), *Reducing Death and Disabilities from Pregnancy and Childbirth* (Port Harcourt, Nigeria: University of Port Harcourt Press, 1990), 37.

5. Federal Ministry of Health, Department of Population Activities, *National Policy on Population for Development, Unity, Progress and Self-Reliance.* (Lagos: Government Printer, 1988), 25.

6. Federal Ministry of Health, *National Policy on Population*, 14.

7. Tola Olu Pearce, *Country Strategy for the Population Program in Nigeria* (report submitted to the MacArthur Foundation, Chicago, 1993).

8. Paulina Makinwa-Adebusoye, *Adolescent Reproductive Behavior in Nigeria.* (Ibadan: Nigerian Institute for Economic and Social Research, monograph no. 3, 1991).

9. John Caldwell, I. O. Orubuloye, and Pat Caldwell, "Fertility Decline in Africa: A New Type of Transition?" *Population and Development Review* 18, no. 2 (1992): 211–42.

10. Tola Olu Pearce, *Women's Reproductive Practices, and Biomedicine: Cultural Conflicts and Transformations* (paper presented at the Wenner-Gren International Conference on The Politics of Reproduction, Brazil, 1991).

11. Pearce, *Women's Reproductive Practices*, 1; Omari Kokole, "The Politics of Fertility in Africa," in *The New Politics of Population*, ed. Jason Finkle and C. Alison McIntosh (New York: The Population Council, 1994), 73–88.

12. National Population Bureau, *The Nigerian Fertility Survey 1981–2* (Lagos: Government Printer, 1984), 14.

13. Betsy Hartmann, *Reproductive Rights and Wrongs* (New York: Harper and Row, 1987), 161–207.

14. Workshop discussions at Northwestern University (Winter Quarter Seminar on *The Politics of Reproduction and Fertility Control in Africa*, Program of African Studies, March 5–6, 1993).

15. Remi Agunlejika, "Primary Health Care and the Child: Professional Nursing Experience in the Ife/Ijisa Zone of Nigeria" in *Child Health in Nigeria*, ed. Tola Olu Pearce and Toyin Falola (Aldershot, England: Avebury Publications, 1994), 117–32.

16. Wambui Wa Karanja, "'Outside Wives' and 'Inside Wives' in Nigeria: A Study of Changing Perceptions in Marriage," in *Transformations of African Marriage*, ed. David Parkins and D. Nyamwaya (Manchester: Manchester University Press, 1987), 247–61.

17. Stella Ogbuagu, "Depo-Provera—A Choice or An Imposition on African Women: A Case Study of Depo-Provera Usage in Maiduguri" in *Women and the Family*, ed. Ayesha Imam et al. (Dakar, Senegal: Codesria, 1985), 122–39; Hartmann, *Reproductive Rights and Wrongs,* 168–73; Pearce, *Women's Reproductive Practices,* 10–11; Ruth Dixon-Mueller, *Population Policy and Women's Rights* (Westport, Conn.: Praeges, 1993), 31–53.

18. Tola Olu Pearce, "Health and Reproduction: Monitoring the Impact of Contraceptive Technology on Women in Nigeria," in *African Women South of the Sahara*, ed. Jean Hay and Sharon Stichter (Essex: Longman, forthcoming).

19. Barbara Mensch et al., "Using Situational Analysis Data to Assess the Functioning of Family Planning Clinics in Nigeria, Tanzania and Zimbabwe," *Studies in Family Planning* 25, no. 1 (1944): 28.

20. Mensch et al., "Using Situational Analysis," 23.

21. Dixon-Mueller, *Population Policy and Women's Rights,* 48.

22. Andrew Abbot, *The System of Professionals* (Chicago: University of Chicago Press, 1991).

23. Ivan Illich, *Medical Nemesis* (London: Boyars, 1969); D. Berman, *The Role of Law in Population Planning* (New York: Oceana, 1972); Vicente Navarro, *Medicine Under Capitalism* (New York: Prodist, 1978); Eliot Freidson, "Are Professionals Necessary?" in *The Authority of Experts*, ed. Thomas Haskell (Bloomington: University of Indiana Press, 1984), 3–27.

24. Bruce Jennings, Daniel Callahan, and Susan Wolf, "The Professions: Public Interest and Common Good," *Hastings Center Report*, Special Supplement (February 1987): 3–10.

25. Jennings, Callahan and Wolf, "The Professions," 6.

26. A. Sesan Ayodele, "Nigeria's Policies and Processes: An Overview," in *Health Research and Health Policy in Nigeria*, ed. Olayiwola Erinosho, John Ohiorhenuan, and Fidelis Ogwumike (lbadan: Adebanke Commercial Press, 1993), 22–23.

27. Ayodele, "Nigeria's Policies," 25.

28. Tola Olu Pearce, "Nigeria's National Health Policy in Perspective: The Scope of Participation" in *Health Research and Health Policy in Nigeria*, ed. Olayiwola Erinosho, John Ohiorhenuan, and Fidelis Ogwumike (lbadan: Adebanke Commercial Press, 1993), 85–93.

29. Dele Olowu, "Local Institutions and Development: The African Experience," *Canadian Journal of African Studies* 23, no. 2 (1989), 201–31.

30. Ade Adetoro, *Patients' Perceptions of the Primary Health Care Program on Ondo State* (M.S. thesis, Obafemi Awolowo University, Ile-Ife, Nigeria, 1989); A. Abasiekong, interview by author, discussant at workshop on Maternal and Childcare in Nigeria, April 1990. Ms. Abasiekong is a nurse by training and an employee of UNICEF (Nigeria).

31. Jennings, Callahan, and Wolf, "The Professions," 6.

32. Sylvester Ogoh Alubo, "Debt Crisis, Health and Health Services in Africa," *Social Science and Medicine* 31, no. 6 (1990): 639–48.

33. O. Akinkugbe, D. Olatunbosum, and G. Esan, eds., *Priorities in National Health Planning* (Ibadan, Nigeria: Caxton Press, 1973) 110–18; Tola Olu Pearce, "Equality of Access to Medical Care: A Review of Nigeria's Approach to Health Promotion," *Ife Social Science Review* F, no. 1 (1985): 156–166; Alubo, "Debt Crisis," 642; Dennis It-yarvar, "Capitalism and Contemporary Forms of Child Abuse," in *Child Health in Nigeria*, ed. Tola Olu Pearce and Toyin Falola (Aldershot, England: Avebury Publications, 1994), 33–43.

34. Workshop discussions at Northwestern University, March 5–6, 1993.

35. Robert Schwartz and Andrew Grubb, "Why Britain Can't Afford Informed Consent," *Hastings Center Report* 15, no. 4 (1985): 19–25.

36. Schwartz and Grubb, "Why Britain Can't Afford Informed Consent," 22.

37. Nicholas Christakis, "The Ethical Design of an AIDS Vaccine in Africa," *Hastings Center Report* 18, no. 3 (1988): 31–37.

38. Tola Olu Pearce, *Importing the New Reproductive Technologies: The Impact of Underlying Models of the Family, Females and Women's Bodies in Nigeria* (paper presented at WIDER Conference on Women, Equality, and Reproductive Technology, Helsinki, Finland, 1992).

39. O. O. Ajayi, "Taboos and Clinical Research in West Africa," *Journal of Medical Ethics* 6, no. 1 (1980): 61–63.

40. Carel Ijsselmuiden and Ruth Faden, "Research and Informed Consent in Africa—Another Look," *New England Journal of Medicine* 326, no. 16 (1992): 830–33.

41. Ijsselmuiden and Faden, "Research and Informed Consent," 833.

42. Wole Soyinka, "Twice Bitten: The Fate of Africa's Cultural Products," in *Challenges of Leadership in African Development*, ed. Olusegun Obasanjo and H. d'Orville (New York: Crane Russak, 1990), 153–68.

43. Ebun Ekunwe and Ross Kessel, "Informed Consent in the Developing World," *Hastings Center Report* 14, no. 3 (1986): 22–24.

44. Bonnie Mass, "An Historical Sketch of the American Population Control Movement," in *Imperialism, Health and Medicine*, ed. Vicente Navarro (New York: Baywood, 1980), 179–202; L. Bondestram and S. Bergstrom, eds., *Poverty and Popula-*

tion Control (London: Academic Press, 1980); John C. Caldwell and Pat Caldwell, "The Cultural Context of High Fertility in Sub-Saharan Africa," *Population and Development Review* 13, no. 3 (1987): 409–37; Paul Erhlich, *The Population Bomb* (New York: Ballantine Books, 1990); Gavin Williams, "The World Bank, Population Control, and the African Environment," *Sociological Review* 4, no. 2 (1992): 3–29.

45. Julian Simon, "The Unreported Revolution in Population Economics," *The Public Interest*, no. 101 (1990): 89.

46. Agnes Riedmann, *Science That Colonizes*, (Philadelphia: Temple University Press, 1993), 2.

47. Riedmann, *Science That Colonizes*, 2.

48. Alubo, "Debt Crisis," 642.

Ellen Hardy

Long-Acting Contraception in Brazil and the Dominican Republic

This paper addresses some situations in which ethical problems may arise with the use of long-acting contraceptive methods in developing countries and mainly presents the author's personal experiences in Brazil and the Dominican Republic.

A method will be considered long-acting if, with a single medical intervention, a woman is protected from pregnancy for at least one menstrual cycle. The discussion will therefore refer to IUDs, subcutaneous implants, injectables, and female sterilization.

The concept of long-acting methods of birth control was developed in the 1960s. Originally these methods were meant to offer unique advantages, such as prolonged contraception for a variable number of years—with the patient making only one decision—and very high efficacy independent of constant individual and/or medical control.[1] Another advantage is that these methods would help prevent involuntary discontinuation that occurs, for example, when women cannot afford to buy oral contraceptives every month or forget their diaphragms at home when they go on vacation.

Nevertheless, practical application of these methods over time has shown that their advantages can also be a source of ethical problems. In developing countries, where contraceptive research and family planning efforts often lack the political and financial support of governments, and where access to adequate health information and health care is limited, there is the possibility of ethical conflict between the desire to offer these methods and the responsibility to protect women from potential abuse.

For this presentation, reference will be made to the following four areas in which ethically complex situations may arise: research, marketing, dependency on health providers, and social control.

Research

For many years, different types of research on contraceptive methods have been carried out in developing countries: basic research, clinical research, introductory trials, and users' perspective studies. For research to be ethical it must be based on a quality proposal and be correctly implemented; subjects must also be well-informed volunteers.

Proposals are usually considered good if prepared by scientists with writing skills who work in developed countries for well-known national or international organizations. These scientists decide what will be studied and how this will be done, and they expect their methodology to be followed rigorously. However, foreign-study designs are flawed when they fail to incorporate the cultural characteristics of the research sites and do not accurately consider the extent of local resources.

Another weakness of these proposals is that they are always written in English, and all collaborating principal investigators are expected to be fluent in this language. Unfortunately, investigators sometimes lack strong language skills and may not have a comprehensive understanding of the proposal or of their discussions with the foreign scientists.

Because local researchers are often not consulted during the planning stage to help identify and propose solutions to potential problems, unexpected difficulties are often encountered during the execution of the project. Among the causes of foreseeable problems are understaffing because of maternity or sick leave, vacation, absences for conferences and staff mobility, strikes of health personnel or transportation workers, and electricity cuts and lack of running water during working hours.

An example of a poor quality research proposal prepared by staff from an international organization follows. Seven developing countries carried out a multicenter study on injectable contraceptives. The proposals and forms were similar but not identical for every country. Training of the research team was mentioned in one proposal, subject selection criteria were not clearly defined in any of them, and a time schedule was presented in just one. Forms were written in the local language in two proposals, and only one included instructions on how to complete the forms. In six proposals some kind of supervision was planned, and instructions on how to manage subjects lost to follow-up were included. Analysis of data was to be carried out by an international organization according to four proposals and by a local institution according to one. Only two proposals mentioned which variables would be studied.

During the implementation process, different problems may occur. Local investigators usually have little or no training in research methodology and are not aware of the need to carefully follow every step of the proposal. For example, in a study to evaluate the effects of three different contraceptives on breast-feeding, only the acceptors of one method were told about the purpose of the study. Women in the other two groups were not. This knowledge or lack of knowledge probably influenced the participants' responses.

In addition, even when local investigators have a good handle on methodology, they are often very busy teaching, seeing patients in the hospital, and working in private practice. Consequently, they must rely on the clinical staff to carry out most of the tasks of the study and do not have time to supervise the work they delegate. The clinical staff is responsible for counselling, providing contraceptive methods, and collecting data.

Another difficulty sometimes encountered during study implementation is improper subject selection. For example, in one study only women who were breast-feeding their babies exclusively or at the most also giving them water or tea, could be included as subjects. It was later found that one local investigator had admitted women who fed their babies "porridge," for he thought it could be considered equivalent to water and tea.

Another example of not following selection criteria can be observed in studies of IUDs, subdermal implants, and injectables. Women should be allowed to enter a study and start using one of these methods only when they are in the first five days of their cycle. This timing helps confirm that the subjects are not pregnant. However, in the introductory trial of Norplant carried out in Brazil, for example, several pregnant women had the implants inserted.

In projects designed abroad, filling out the interview forms for each subject is another potential source of error that can affect the study results. These forms are designed for computerized reading and are printed on "auto-copy" paper which is rarely found in developing countries. Since it is nearly impossible to preserve the format during translation and to obtain the right paper, local researchers are forced to use forms in English. The reason for this is that sometimes they are not allowed to prepare a form in the local language and later transcribe the information to the form in English, because this could produce errors. Staff members with variable English language skills obtain the required information by questioning the patients in the local language and then checking the appropriate box on the form. Other problems with the forms may be that the questions are directed to the interviewer rather than to the subject or that there is a list of items for which information must be obtained. In the latter case each staff member will probably word the questions differently. Clearly, accuracy is jeopardized with this complex procedure.

Another possible problem is that regular follow-up of subjects may not be achieved because they postpone, miss, or never attend their appointments. This may happen because they don't have money for public transportation, have family obligations, or cannot be absent from work. Some women actually move to another city or country, even though they were told that admission to the study required local residence. This was a problem in the Dominican Republic, where some Norplant implant users emigrated to the United States.

When patients are lost to follow-up in studies on long-term methods, there is a negative impact on both the study results and, potentially, on the health of women. In the case of injectables, the researchers can assume that a woman was subject to the effects of the drug until its complete excretion; however, with IUDs and subcutaneous implants there is no way of knowing how long they were used. For all these methods, the reasons for discontinuation will never be known. Nor will the reasons women suffered any ill health effects.

An additional source of difficulty involves informed consent. An informed consent is a required part of a research proposal that should explain the study in a way that helps a woman decide if she wants to volunteer. Nevertheless, detailed information does not guarantee that women will understand what a study is and that participation involves acceptance of certain risks, benefits, and responsibilities. A problem in using a written informed consent is that this text is often not read or understood by the women. A long text presented orally requires continued attention, and often women sign in trust without having heard or read all the content.

Even if an adequate informed consent is attained, it does not guarantee voluntarism when the method being studied is the only one offered. For example, in one study in which women had to choose between three contraceptive methods, a local investigator offered only one of them at a time until he had completed the required number of acceptors for each method.

Suggestions for Improvement

It is necessary to improve the quality of the study proposals designed to be conducted in developing countries. First, investigators from these countries must be involved from the beginning so that their ideas are incorporated as the proposal develops. This will allow them to understand more clearly their responsibilities and to express their concerns about future difficulties. The experience will improve their knowledge of research methodology, ethical issues, and their counselling skills.

In order that new methods of contraception introduced into developing countries serve the needs of women, it is important that social scientists contribute to the preparation and implementation of research proposals. Their knowledge and experience will help to prevent unexpected problems. In addition, sufficient funds should be made available to ensure appropriate supervision and follow-up of projects. Continuous supervision is needed at all levels so that mistakes are corrected as soon as possible.

Study implementation also needs improvement. Local researchers should be trained in research methodology, including ethical considerations and counselling skills. The proposal and forms should be translated into the local language and made available to the whole staff. The need to follow the proposal carefully and to fill out the forms correctly must be emphasized.

Therefore, principal investigators must involve and train the whole research team. Its members need to be told about the purpose of the study and must have information on methodology specific to the project. Furthermore, they must learn how to carry out interviews, complete forms, and be given instructions on what to do when a subject misses an appointment. Care must be taken not to overburden staff with long working hours or with activities for which they are unprepared or not remunerated.[2]

Voluntary participation must be ensured. Informed consent should be obtained in culturally appropriate ways. It will not always be necessary to have signed statements of consent because women may be suspicious when asked to sign if they have never done so when obtaining health services. The largest possible variety of contraceptives should be available, and good counselling should be provided so that women choose freely among methods and truly volunteer for study participation. Staff that provides counselling should be trained and supervised.

Finally, those lost to follow-up problem must be dealt with. If the need to locate a woman in the field should arise, it is crucial to have obtained correct information on where she lives. When women have volunteered to participate they must be told of the importance of follow-up, since this may enhance compliance with scheduled visits to the clinic. Consequently, when women are included in the study their addresses should be recorded in detail.[3] Funds will be needed for field visits that are expensive and very time-consuming.

Marketing and Distribution

In many developing countries, when a contraceptive becomes available on the market, control of its distribution is usually lacking or inadequate. Anyone can buy it. The most prescribed methods are those that allow more profit making. Providers are often insufficiently trained in the provision of these methods and do not have counselling skills or a solid understanding of the ethical aspects of use.

In one country, during the 1960s, physicians working for the public health service were paid for each IUD they inserted. This encouraged the use of the method. When the physician incentives were discontinued, the rate of use decreased and IUDs were generally offered only upon request. Some physicians

TABLE 1.   Percent distribution by region of women fifteen to forty-four years old using different contraceptive methods. 1986

Method	Total	RJ	SP	South	BH/ES	North East	North
Tubal Ligation	41.6	47.5	43.3	25.2	40.1	47.8	66.7
Pills	38.2	35.6	34.0	54.6	37.5	32.8	21.3
Other	20.2	16.9	22.6	20.3	22.0	19.9	12.5

RJ   -Rio de Janeiro
SP   -São Paulo
BH/ES   -Belo Horizonte/Espírito Santo

Source: Data from J. M. Arruda, N. Rutemberg, L. Morris, E. A. Ferraz. Pesquisa Nacional sobre Saúde Materno-Infantil e Planejamiento Familiar (National study on maternal-child health and family planning) (bound report, BEMFAM, Rio de Janeiro, Brazil, December, 1987), 66.

went so far as to remove IUDs they had been paid to insert without telling the women.

Another example of this misuse involves tubal ligation in Brazil (table 1), the method used by the largest percentage of women.[4] In this country most women, if counselled about the procedure at all, receive incomplete information. They are not given a description of the surgical procedure and often do not understand that they should consider the method irreversible. There are women who believe tubal ligation lasts five years or that the "knots" can be untied at any time. At one university's infertility clinic, between 1978 and 1980, 2.4% of the women requesting treatment were infertile secondary to a tubal ligation. This percentage increased to 12.4% from 1988 to 1990. Of 165 women who underwent a laparoscopy to determine potential for reversal, nearly half (46.7%) were found to be without a chance.

Results from a Brazilian study on women's health issues showed that the main factor associated with being sterilized before the age of twenty-five was familiarity with a smaller number of contraceptive methods. This is a clear indication that the attending physicians do not always offer alternative means of fertility regulation before carrying out the irreversible procedure of tubal ligation. We emphasized surgical sterilization before the age of twenty-five, because other studies have shown that about half of the women who had a tubal ligation that young will regret having done so a few years later.

Because this surgery is considered illegal in the country, physicians tend to perform tubal ligations as an adjunct to another primary procedure such as a Caesarean section. This association of procedures results in many unnecessary c-sections, with physicians being paid under the table even when a woman has health insurance or is in a public or philanthropic hospital.

TABLE 2.   Percentage of women who had a Caesarean section in order to be sterilized.

							Total
Regret	Cases	67.6	216	Controls	60.6	216	64.1
Paism 1	São Paulo	42.1	375	Interior	31.2	436	36.3

Source: E. Hardy, data from the following study: "Arrependimento após a esterilização cirúrgica. Estudo caso-controle" (Regret After Sterilization. A Case-Control Study), 1993.
E. Hardy, data from the following study: "Avalição do programa de assistência integral à saúde da mulher no Estado de São Paulo" (Evaluation of the Program for Women's Integral Health Care in São Paulo State), 1988.

In a recent Brazilian study on sterilization regret, subjects were asked whether they had the tubal ligation during a Caesarean section.[5] Interim results show that 64.1% of all the women interviewed responded affirmatively (table 2). The aforementioned study that addressed women's health issues also found that among subjects who had a tubal ligation, half were sterilized at the same time that they had a Caesarean section (table 2).

Another profit-driven method in Brazil is Norplant implants. Lately, this contraceptive has been offered to physicians by a firm that imports pharmaceuticals. When company representatives were asked over the phone whether they had a system for training, they answered that it is not necessary to train buyers to insert and remove the implants because written instructions are provided. These instructions—for buyers and users—are all in English.

An additional example of unethical marketing of contraceptives in Latin America involves a monthly injectable, dihydroxyprogesterone acetophenide. This injection was removed from the market in Europe in the 1960s, and the results from animal studies requested by the FDA for approval in the United States were never reported by the manufacturer. In spite of the doubtful or negative toxicology that precluded the use of the method in the developed world, the same product has been marketed since the 1980s in the region, where regulations are weak and approval easier to be obtain.

Suggestions for Improvement

Long-term contraceptive methods should be introduced under controlled conditions. Providers should receive high-quality theoretical and practical training. In the case of IUDs and subcutaneous implants, this training would include practice of both insertion and removal. Sales should be restricted to trained health professionals, and control mechanisms should be established. For example, in the Dominican Republic, Norplant implants can only be bought from PROFAMILIA, IPPF's affiliate. The method is only sold to

TABLE 3. Percent distribution of former Norplant users according to how long they had to wait to have the implants removed. Dominican Republic.

	Clinic			
Waited	*A*	*B*	*C*	*Total*
Did not wait	65	40	28	44.0
Up to 1 week	26	29	31	28.4
8 days–3 months	9	31	41	27.3
Total women	31	48	29	109

Source: Data from E. Hardy, C. Baez, T. Rodrigues, et al., "Users' attitudes about Norplant contraceptives subdermal implants and changes that occur with use of the method. Report of answers to pre-coded questions. Dominican Republic" (bound report, CEMICAMP, Campinas, Brazil, December 1987), 128.

physicians who were trained at the PROFAMILIA clinic, and the institution keeps an updated list of their names.

Dependency on Health Providers

All long-acting contraceptives require health care intervention for initiation. This varies from giving an injection to performing tubal ligations. Provider intervention is also required for discontinuation of IUDs and subcutaneous implants—and even more so for reversal of sterilization. The fulfillment of a woman's decision to initiate or to discontinue use depends on the availability and willingness of trained health professionals. This limits a woman's power to make her own decisions about use and favors the imposition of continued use.

A user's perspective study of Norplant implant acceptors was carried out in the Dominican Republic. Current users and 109 women who had discontinued use were interviewed. The latter were questioned about their experiences with removal. Less than half of the women obtained removal on the day of their request (table 3).

Subjects were also asked about the reasons for removal delay. Half the women said they had arrived late at the clinic or had been informed that an appointment was required for removal. The second most frequently mentioned reason for delay was that their request for removal was initially determined to be irrelevant (table 4).

Suggestions for Improvement

Since dependency on health care providers cannot be avoided, steps must be taken to ensure that access to providers and counselling is never restricted. At the same time, a woman's decision to use or discontinue a method after

Table 4. Percent distribution of former Norplant users according to reasons for not having the implants removed the same day requested. Dominican Republic.

Reason	Clinic			
	A	B	C	Total
Late/appointment needed	36	65	38	51
Removal refused*	54	17	24	26
Continuation suggested	18	3	19	11
Other	—	17	38	21
Total women	11	29	21	61

* A/B p<.02

she has received counselling needs to be respected. This should occur even if the health provider thinks that the woman has chosen the "wrong" method or wants to discontinue for an "irrelevant" reason.

The pace of introduction should not exceed the system's capacity to provide removal, even though this will mean denying the method to some women. Finally, economic incentives to use a specific method should be avoided.

Social Control

When discussing the social control of research and the marketing of long-acting contraceptives, the following should be considered: control is partly carried out by the mass media, but the information it provides is ambiguous and equivocal; organized women's groups have a unique role to play, but radical and/or poorly informed feminist groups have a negative effect on women's choice; the medical establishment has weak internal ethical control.

Information on contraceptives is uncritically accepted by the mass media and published according to the journalistic concept of news. A new method makes the headlines if it is considered a breakthrough, and any method makes the headlines if it is thought to cause terrible side effects. This has been the case in Brazil with Norplant implants. It was initially described on television and in the written media as a very good method. Later, without any confirmation, news organizations accused the university where the research had been carried out of harming women through the use of Norplant.

In developing countries, especially in Brazil, organized women's groups are the main force promoting social control of contraceptive research and marketing. The problem is that they tend to endorse or veto specific methods such as the diaphragm and Norplant, respectively. Radical and/or poorly informed groups do not consider the consequences of disseminating incorrect, frightening information about methods such as IUDs and Norplant. Women using these contraceptives have been unnecessarily distressed by this information, and a large number have subsequently requested discontinuation. Ironically, this feminist effort leads to fewer contraceptive options for women.

The medical establishment's concerns frequently are limited to the protection of health professionals and not of clients. Physicians rationalize unethical procedures. This is reflected, for example, in the 90–95% rate of Caesarean sections among private patients in Brazil. Usually, women are then sterilized after the third baby. In addition, Caesarean sections are frequently done with the sole purpose of providing sterilization.

Suggestions for Improvement

Social control must be improved so that it is valid and useful. Researchers and health professionals should actively provide journalists with correct information before and during the introduction of a method. This should ensure the dissemination of factual information in the media, which should better serve the needs and interests of women. Women's groups and the medical establishment should work to promote constructive dialogue between women's health advocates and contraceptive researchers and providers.

Conclusions

When international funding organizations design study proposals, they must accept the responsibilities that accompany authorship. First, they must write quality proposals and ensure that these are correctly implemented. This requires consultation with local researchers and social scientists during the planning phase and the provision of adequate supervision at the site. Second, they have to understand that research efforts in developing countries often require substantial financial support and time allowances, and they must be prepared to provide for these needs.

Poor quality proposals and incorrectly implemented studies based on adequate proposals both result in inaccurate and potentially harmful findings. Even though subjects may not experience any health problems as a result of their participation in a poor study, their valuable time and energy investments are wasted. If researchers ask their subjects to take their participation responsibly, they in turn must respect this commitment. Also, women in general can be affected by results from poor studies, since policies will be based on this information.

Once a woman has received the best possible counselling, considering the local counselling resources, her decision about which method to use and her reason for requesting removal should be respected. Final responsibility for these decisions should usually rest with each woman and not with the health providers.

It will probably be years before the large-scale and proper use of reversible long-acting contraceptives is established in Brazil. In the meantime, surgeons should perform tubal ligations in a way that allows for the best chance for reversal, since a number of women will inevitably regret having had the surgery.

NOTES

1. Conselho Estadual da Condição Feminina. "O direito de ter ou não ter filhos no Brasil" (The right to have or not to have children in Brazil) *Cadernos* 1 (1986), 23–24.

2. J. G. Cleland, E. E. Hardy, E. Taucher, *Introduction of New Contraceptives into Family Planning Programmes* (Geneva: The World Health Organization, 1990), 67.

3. Ibid.

4. J. M. Arruda, N. Rutemberg, L. Morris, E. A. Ferraz, Pesquisa Nacional sobre Saúde Materno-Infantil e Planejamento Familiar, Brasil (1986) (National study on maternal-child health and family planning) (BEMFAM, Rio de Janeiro, Brazil, December 1987), 66.

5. E. Hardy, data from the following study, "Arrependimento após a esterilização cirúrgica. Estudo caso-controle" (Regret after sterilization. A case-control study) (CEMICAMP, Campinas, Brazil, September 1993).

Contributors

JOHN D. ARRAS is the Porterfield Professor of Biomedical Ethics in the Department of Philosophy at the University of Virginia, Charlottesville, Virginia.

JEFFREY BLUSTEIN is an associate professor in the Division of Bioethics of the Department of Epidemiology and Social Medicine at Montefiore Medical Center/Albert Einstein College of Medicine, Bronx, New York.

GEORGE F. BROWN is vice president, Programs Division, of The Population Council, New York, New York.

DANIEL CALLAHAN is president of The Hastings Center, Briarcliff Manor, New York.

REBECCA DRESSER is a professor at the School of Law and the Center for Biomedical Ethics, Case Western Reserve University, Cleveland, Ohio.

ELLEN HARDY is an assistant professor in the Department of Obstetrics and Gynecology at the Faculty of Medical Sciences, Universidade Estadual de Campinas, Campinas, São Paulo, Brazil.

BRUCE JENNINGS is executive director of The Hastings Center, Briarcliff Manor, New York.

RUTH MACKLIN is a professor in the Division of Philosophy and History of Medicine of the Department of Epidemiology and Social Medicine at Montefiore Medical Center/Albert Einstein College of Medicine, Bronx, New York.

ELLEN H. MOSKOWITZ is associate for law at The Hastings Center, Briarcliff Manor, New York.

HILDE LINDEMANN NELSON is director of the Center for Applied and Professional Ethics at the University of Tennessee, Knoxville, Tennessee.

JAMES LINDEMANN NELSON is a professor of philosophy at the University of Tennessee, Knoxville, Tennessee.

TOLA OLU PEARCE is an associate professor in the Department of Sociology and the Women's Studies Program at the University of Missouri, Columbia, Missouri.

KATHLEEN E. POWDERLY is assistant director of the Division of Humanities in Medicine, and assistant professor of nursing and obstetrics and gynecology at the State University of New York Health Science Center, Brooklyn, New York.

JOHN A. ROBERTSON holds the Vinson and Elkins Chair at the University of Texas School of Law at Austin.

BONNIE STEINBOCK is a professor of philosophy at the University at Albany/SUNY, Albany, New York.

Index